F*CK FIBROMYALGIA

A Simple Step by Step Breakdown: Natural Treatment Protocols toward Ultimate Remission.

Earth Doctor Organics

This book is dedicated to all the women and men suffering from chronic pain.

My hope is to provide every Fibromyalgia patient with simple, affordable research based insights towards regaining freedom from this menacing and often silent medical condition. You are not alone!!

The material has been written and published for educational purposes only. The reader understands that the author is not engaged in rendering medical advice or services via this text. The author provides this information, and the reader accepts it with the understanding that people act at their own risk and with full knowledge that they should consult with a medical professional for medical help. Although the author and publisher have made every effort to ensure that the information in this book was correct at press time, the author and publisher do not assume and hereby disclaim any liability to any party for any loss, damage, or disruption caused by errors or omissions, whether such errors or omissions result from negligence, accident, or any other cause. The author shall have neither liability nor responsibility to any person, or entity with respect to any loss, damages, or injury caused, or alleged to be caused, directly or indirectly by the information contained in this book.

This book is not intended as a substitute for the medical advice of your individual primary care physician. The reader should regularly consult their doctor in matters relating to his/her health and particularly with respect to any symptoms that may require physical, clinical and laboratory diagnosis or acute medical attention.

The information in this book is meant to supplement, not replace, proper individualized patient centered care. Like any pharmaceutical, exercise, diet and neutraceutical intervention there may be some inherent risks. The authors and publisher advise readers to take full responsibility for their health and safety by speaking to their health care practitioner prior to beginning any treatment protocols.

Before practicing the exercise skills described in this book, be sure that you consult a healthcare practitioner and that equipment is well maintained. Do not take risks beyond your level of experience and aptitude.

FIBROMYALGIA: THE INSIDIOUS CHRONIC CONDITION THAT IS DISABLING MILLIONS.

OVERVIEW

Over the past many years, within my own medical private practice I have come across an unprecedented number of patients reporting abnormally elevated sensitivity to pain. At the same time, many of these fibromyalgic patients are also experiencing other chief concerns beyond widespread chronic muscle and joint discomfort. This often explains their health history of clinical confusion and misdiagnosis.

Listed below are ten of the many random complaints my Fibromyalgia patients have reported to me:

1. Myalgia (Unrelenting muscle ache throughout the body with increased sensitivity and pain when touched; sometimes associated with morning joint stiffness)

2. Irritable Bowel Syndrome (passing alternating hard to liquid stool; gas and bloating with abdominal discomfort; sensitivity to various foods, especially gluten or wheat based products)

3. Chronic Fatigue (Low energy throughout the day; difficulty initiating sleep while also feeling unrested upon waking; often experiencing mid-afternoon sleepiness with intense caffeine or sugar cravings)

4. Headaches (intermittent or chronic tension headaches; sometimes with dizziness and light sen-

sitivity/photophobia)

5. Dysmenorrhea (painful periods consisting of intense menstrual cramping)

6. Weight Loss Resistance (An inability to lose weight despite dietary caloric restriction and a consistent exercise regimen)

7. Jaw Pain (Sometimes presenting with stress and headaches; often related to 'bruxism' which is an abnormal grinding or clenching of the teeth)

8. Cognitive Dysfunction (Feeling "hazy" or "foggy" with memory; difficulty concentrating on tasks and poor verbal recall)

9. Neuralgia (Nerve Pain which may present as burning, stabbing, numbness or tingling in the body)

10. Skin Abnormalities (Sensitive skin that is reactive to temperature changes; which may at times present with a rash or reaction to various chemicals in daily cosmetic products)

According to research published by The American College of Rheumatology, Fibromyalgia now affects up to 8% of the population making it one of the top diagnosed rheumatic disorders[1]. However, despite increased recognition of this disabling and chronic condition it has been estimated that millions of sufferers are still undiagnosed[2].

So, why is there such discrepancy in diagnosis?

Perhaps it is due to the poor medical diagnostic

and testing criteria for Fibromyalgia. Alternatively, it may also be due to the fact that this disorder often presents with so many varied symptoms; which tend to mimic a long list of other health disorders and pathologies.

The implications of this are significant!

Many Fibromyalgia patients are suffering from chronic pain that greatly disables their ability to engage in even the most basic activities of daily living. Some activities that may be compromised include physical movement (cooking, cleaning, exercising), job performance and more significantly, social relationships with family and friends[3]. Subsequently, this can result in low mood and an overall poor quality of life for fibromyalgia syndrome patients.

As a Naturopathic Doctor, it is important to admit that diagnosis and effective natural treatment avenues for Fibromyalgia have been very difficult to achieve over the years. I have seen firsthand the exacerbated stress among patients struggling to legitimize a diagnosis and garner support through the health care system. This is ultimately one of the main reasons I decided to write this book; as this chronic disabling disorder is also a great economic drain on patients and social healthcare as a whole[4].

MY STORY

Pain can change a person. At the beginning of my medical career I used to be a very active, positive and joyful individual. I thrived through happy relationships with family and friends. I was passionately dedicated to spending long hours cultivating health among my amazing patients within my private practice.

Then one beautiful summer morning while I was stopped at a red light, I was struck by a distracted driver who was speeding while on his cell phone. A year of the worst pain I'd ever experienced followed. These dark days consisted of a concussion followed by post-concussion syndrome; herniated spinal discs that impinged the nerve roots in my neck and sent shooting pain into my back; a broken right hand with ligament tears; and a muscle tear in my right knee that caused instability and swelling. The whiplash, combined with the brain injury created nausea, mood changes and irrational anxiety and severely negative thought cycles.

I began pharmaceuticals immediately. I saw the best therapists, doctors and specialists; doing everything I could to expedite my healing.

One year later, my energy was at an all time low, while my pain was at an all time high. At this point even walking down the aisle at the grocery store became unbearable. I had constant stiffness and pain in my joints. My mood alternated between angry and sad. I was overweight and unable to shed the pounds. I even developed irritable bowel disease.

Most significantly, at any point I felt like I would lose my mind having to endure the constant burning in my back and sore tender muscles throughout my body. I could not tolerate exercise, let alone engage mentally, physically and emotionally in my relationships or career. My mind was foggy and I became unrecognizably pessimistic. I did not connect with my romantic partner. Worst of all, I could not stand to be touched-even a hug would send me spiralling in pain.

My family doctor then confirmed a diagnosis of fibromyalgia. Years later I often see fibromyalgia onset in patients who have a history of car accidents or other forms of sudden and intense stress in their lives.

During one of the many nights of frequent insomnia, in between tears of painful discomfort and frustration, I vowed to find an effective and alternative treatment protocol to target Fibromyalgia and return the body and mind to functional health.

Throughout this text, we will focus on getting rid of pain, clearing the "brain fog"; losing weight, gastrointestinal health as well as, boosting energy and mood. I hope the contents in this text will help demystify the illness and help you heal and progress to remission from fibromyalgia.

This book will provide an effective fibromyalgia

protocol that has taken many years of clinical practice and self-care to fine tune. It has helped not only me, but many patients too. Included here, you will find key naturopathic fibromyalgia treatment protocols. This book will also include details on blood work, supplements, acupuncture points, dietary interventions and much more.

The information presented is used daily within my integrative medical practice and can be fine tuned to fit your symptoms, lifestyle and physical abilities. I hope you will also share the information presented here with your health care practitioner. It is purposeful in targeting the root cause of fibromyalgic illness and treating the whole person, not only the individual symptoms.

It is my goal here to arm each fibromyalgia patient with an easy arsenal of evidence based medical treatment options with which we can target flare ups, as well as completely eradicate fibromyalgia syndrome. –Earth Doctor

CURRENT SCIENTIFIC RESEARCH AND THEORIES.

WHAT CAUSES FIBROMYAGLIA?

The root cause of fibromyalgia has been debated for years within the scientific medical community. Despite the controversy, there is still no definitive known cause. However, ongoing research has put forth new insights and evolving theories. These all contribute to better conventional drug and alternative medicine treatment approaches.

Fibromyalgia manifests as an abnormally increased pain sensitivity and lowered pain tolerance among sufferers[5]. Why does this happen? Why does Lucy tolerate and enjoy her weekly massage at the spa; when Susan who suffers from fibromyalgia, finds the pressure on her tender muscles to be torturous and increasingly painful?

Susan exhibits something called "central nervous system sensitization". Her chronic pain over time may have changed how her nervous system functions. This modification in the brain renders her even more hypersensitive to painful triggers. She may even react negatively to things that she previously was able to tolerate. We can actually track the abnormal processing of pain in the brains of fibromyalgia patients like Susan, through a MRI[6].

The following section of the book will explore the causal factors of this illness. I will try my best to simplify the scientific jargon here. However, there are some key concepts regarding brain centers, hormones and nerve pathways that I must detail for your consideration.

This information will enable you to better understand how the fibromyalgia treatment options (presented later in this book) work.

LOW SEROTONIN HYPOTHESIS

You may have heard of serotonin (also known as 5-hydroxytryptamine or 5-HT) often referred to as the "happy" hormone. Serotonin is a "neurotransmitter". A neurotransmitter is a substance used by the nerves in our body to signal and communicate with each other. It plays a role in regulating our brains' behaviour. Serotonin is implicated in mood, memory, learning, sleep and even sexual desire[7].

90% of serotonin in the body is located in the gastrointestinal (GI) tract where it helps regulate gut motor activity[8]. Serotonin also plays a role in **pain regulation**, also known as "**nociceptive regulation**" within the body[5]. The "low serotonin" or "serotonin deficiency" theory hypothesizes that fibromyalgia syndrome patients have a decreased amount of serotonin in the central nervous system (brainstem and spinal cord)[9]. Researchers proposed that this lack of serotonin messes with the pain reduction or pain blocking mechanisms in the central nervous system, rendering these pathways less effective[6]. Here, the low serotonin is believed to result in an abnormal pain response or an increased pain perception to an otherwise tolerable or normal incoming sensory input[6].

A scientific study published in the *Journal of Rheumatology* noted that when blood samples from fibromyalgia syndrome patients were analyzed, lower levels of serotonin were found in comparison to healthy people[10].

Lower levels of the amino acid tryptophan have also been found in the blood of fibromyalgia syndrome patients in comparison to healthy subjects[11]. This is significant as tryptophan is converted into serotonin in the body. Furthermore, serotonin in turn is needed to make melatonin, a hormone that regulates sleep and wakefulness. Perhaps low serotonin decreases melatonin production which may account for all the sleep issues that arise in fibromyalgia.

In another experiment, researchers measured the cerebrospinal fluid of patients with fibromyalgia syndrome, the biomarkers of serotonin present in the brain and spine were again found to be at a level lower than normal[12]. The above theory would explain why healthy individuals can tolerate wearing a backpack, receiving a hug and even going for a jog; while fibromyalgia patients find the same physical stimuli intolerable and painful.

On the other hand, there are many scientific studies that challenge the serotonin deficiency theory of fibromyalgia. Scientists in refute of this low-serotonin theory will refer to the short-lived and often weak effect that selective serotonin reuptake inhibitor drugs (SSRIs) have on fibromyalgia symptom relief[13]. These SSRI drugs are anti-depressants that help to increase the amount of serotonin available in the nervous system. It was once thought that since the SSRIs increased serotonin levels at nerve sites in the body, then the symptoms of inappropriate pain response and hypersensitivity should resolve. This is based on the premise that there is now enough serotonin in the SSRI treated fibromyalgia patient to regulate the pain receptors appropriately. However, some researchers have gone as far as to conclude the effects of antidepressants in the treatment of fibromyalgia are no better than placebo[14]. Basically, stating they are ineffective at reducing pain. This is where the controversy arises, because some patients have actually found positive improvement of mood, sleep and pain with SSRI use for fibromyalgia syndrome[15].

It is clear from the conflicting research that serotonin may play an important role in fibromyalgia syndrome. Ultimately, this is only one small component, connected to many other factors which play a role in causing this menacing disease.

LOW METABOLISM THEORY

The Thyroid Connection

The low metabolism theory of fibromyalgia syndrome proposes that an abnormal hypersensitivity to pain (called hyperalgesia) is linked to our thyroid. This pain response may be due to hypothyroidism or a partial resistance to the thyroid hormones that are being produced in the body[16]. This low metabolism theory also explores alternate reasons that could cause chronic pain, such as poor diet causing nutritional deficiencies, poor physical fitness and even drugs that can cause metabolic issues leading to fibromyalgic symptoms[16].

There are two main types of thyroid hormones produced in the body: T3 (Triiodothyronine) and T4 (thyroxine). Of the two, T3 is the most active form. It has been established that about 90% of fibromyalgia patients have thyroid dysfunction to some extent[17].

So you may be reading this and thinking, let's just give everyone suffering from fibromyalgia thyroid hormone therapy. Could it be as simple as that? In some instances, yes it is! Case studies have shown that oral therapy of thyroid hormone (T3) has helped fibromyalgia patients with hypothyroidism (a low-functioning thyroid)[18]. Oral thyroid medication has also been found to improve fibromyalgia symptoms among patients who have a normal functioning thyroid but show signs of cellular resistance to the thyroid hormones they produce[19].

A 5 year study found that fibromyalgia patients who were given thyroid hormone recovered significantly from fibromyalgia syndrome[20]. These patients had hypothyroidism or alternatively, a normal functioning thyroid but signs of thyroid hormone resistance in the body. Later in this book, we will discuss how you and your doctor can figure out if this is a possible therapy route for you. However, it is important to note that these lucky fibromyalgic patients who improved with therapy were also taking nutritional supplements, exercising regularly and eating a wholesome diet. The effects of such metabolism altering lifestyle changes were exemplified in another experiment, where 25% of fibromyalgia patients who did not change their diet or take supplements, found no improvement with thyroid hormone therapy alone[21].

Before moving on, we must discuss the thyroid connection to pain. The chronic muscle tenderness and abnormal pain responses in fibromyalgia syndrome are regulated by the nociceptive (pain) systems in our brainstem and spinal cord. It is here where thyroid hormone plays an interesting role.

The pain sensory nerves (nociceptors) respond to potentially harmful stimuli and signal a warning to the brain via the spinal cord of any possible threat to the body. In fibromyalgia patients, this pain signalling to the brain may be hyperactive. This is due to an excess of something called substance P. Substance P is the main neurotransmitter in the body that signals pain to the brain. The cerebrospinal fluid (the fluid around the brain and spinal cord) of fibromyalgia patients has been shown to contain excessive levels of substance P[22]. Remember, higher substance P levels mean more pain signals are being sent to the brain.

Thyroid hormone normally stops the production and secretion of substance P in the central nervous system[23]. In animal studies, the surgical removal of the thyroid (thyroidectomy) resulted in an increase of substance P levels in various areas of the spine and brain[24]. Alternatively, treatment with thyroid hormone was shown many years ago to lower substance P levels in the brain[24].

Poor thyroid hormone regulation may also stop our anti-nociceptive systems from working properly by reducing the production of norepinephrine in an area of our brainstem called the locus coeruleus[25]. Norepinephrine (or noradrenaline) is a hormone and neurotransmitter found at higher levels in the body during stressful periods. It is made from another neurotransmitter named dopamine. Norepinephrine is incredibly important to the normal functioning of our anti-pain systems[26]. Low markers of dopamine and norepinephrine were found in the brain and spinal fluid of fibromyalgia patients[12]. Studies have also found that the locus coeruleus cells in the brain contain the highest levels of the thyroid hormone T3[27]. Thus, it is hypothesized that in hypothyroid, fibromyalgic patients, the low T3 levels in the locus coeruleus may cause low norepinephrine production, resulting in dysfunctional pain regulation[26].

Additionally, serotonin levels in the central nervous system may depend on the amount of norepinephrine being produced[25]. When there is a normal amount of serotonin being produced, serotonin can increase opiates in the body. These opiates are basically pain reducing substances. Opiates can block the release of substance P as well as another pro-pain substance called glutamate[28].

To recap the above theory, in the most simplified way: A poor thyroid hormone metabolism results in low epinephrine levels in the brainstem, which may reduce serotonin levels, which in turn will reduce opiate secretion. The low thyroid hormone levels slow epinephrine production which will render the anti-nociceptive (anti-pain) pathways in the central nervous system as dysfunctional. Meanwhile the nociceptive (pro-pain) pathways will increase in signalling. This all may lead to an abnormal pain perception among fibromyalgic individuals.

Although these hypo-metabolism and poor thyroid regulation theories have not been affirmed as the official cause of fibromyalgia pain, they would definitely explain a lot of the other symptoms we experience during the disease process. Parallel symptoms of low thyroid hormone include: extreme tiredness, irregular sleep patterns, dry skin, thinning hair, brittle nails, painful periods, cold intolerance, joint pain and stiffness and inadequate stress response.

I wish fibromyalgia syndrome was a simple disease process. Unfortunately, it is incredibly multi-faceted. For the purpose of targeting all the possible factors contributing to your individual experience with fibromyalgia, it is also important to explore genetics, stress and diet.

GENETIC RISK FACTORS IN FIBROMYALGIA

Studies in the field of neuropsychiatry have established that many factors may contribute to an individual becoming susceptible to developing fibromyalgia syndrome[29]. This includes potential genetic risk factors.

Researchers have linked various genes to an increased risk of becoming fibromyalgic. *RGS4* is the name of one of those genes associated with fibromyalgia syndrome[30].

Earlier we talked about a section in the brainstem known as the "locus coeruleus". When this brain area was not well regulated by T3 thyroid hormone it resulted in low norepinephrine production. Interestingly enough, the *RGS4* gene activity also takes place in the locus coeruleus[31]. It is here that this gene has been linked to the down regulation or decrease of opioid receptor functioning[3].

The opioid receptors in our body serve to block pain. So, a decreased availability of these receptors in the brains of fibromyalgia patients sets great implications. We can infer that if less pain blocking (opioid) receptors are available to us, then a decrease in pain reduction and increased pain perception may occur. This may also explain why opioid drugs such as hydrocodone, morphine and even codeine may not provide all fibromyalgia patients with pain relief, as these drugs must bind to the available opioid receptors.

When it comes to chronic pain, fibromyalgia has been found to exist among family members[2]. This genetic link to fibromyalgia syndrome is emphasized in monozygotic twin studies. Monozygotic twins (who share 100% identical genes at birth) were found to have a greater susceptibility of both developing fibromyalgia when compared to siblings groups who shared less identical DNA[32].

Another gene of interest that is currently under investigation is called *COMT* (Catechol-O-methyltransferase)[33]. One genetic variation of this gene, associated with fibromyalgic patients is known as *COMT* val158met [34]. This genetic variant of *COMT* has been linked to higher pain sensitivity[34]. *COMT* val158met has also been linked to psychological distress among fibromyalgia patients[35]. This link between genetics, stress and pain is still being studied in-depth. However, it seems that beyond a foundation of genetics, fibromyalgia pain may be linked to psychological and environmental stressors.

STRESS SUCKS

There is no published medical evidence to specifically prove that fibromyalgia occurs after a negative life event. However, when going through the past decade of my patient research and treatment files, I could not help but see a pattern of physical and emotional trauma prior to the fibromyalgia disease onset.

Was this the trigger to a lifetime of muscular pain and fatigue? Why did some patients develop fibromyalgia under such stressful life conditions, while others were able to cope and reclaim their lives without chronic pain?

Many of these fibromyalgia patients, like me, had experienced a devastating car accident and physical injuries that drastically changed their lives. Others noted the loss of a loved one (including beloved pets), miscarriage and romantic break-ups. Some patients were even diagnosed with fibromyalgia after a bad bout of illness. When looking at health history, I found a surprising number of my fibromyalgia patients had also experienced childhood bullying and sexual/physical abuse. Whereas others noted being unhappy with the performance stress and politics in their workplace for many years. There was even one case, where I had treated a professional hockey player who suffered from repetitive concussions and chronic anxiety only to retire from the sport and battle fibromyalgia for 20 years.

As controversial as it may seem to ask...Are any of these life experiences relevant to the creation of fibromyalgia syndrome? As this book is written with a focus on evidence based medicine-I will utilize the scientific studies available to help us understand how stress can contribute to the initiation, aggravation and exacerbation of fibromyalgia.

When it comes to pain perception, we have established that

it is increased in fibromyalgia. Similarly, fibromyalgic sufferers also have an increased perception of stress, when compared to healthy individuals[36]. This can be exemplified by studies where healthy subjects rated life stressors as "mild"; whereas fibromyalgia subjects rated the same stressors as much worst in severity[37]. When we are unable to cope with stressors in our environment, we become more susceptible to health problems such as depression[37]. If stress plays a significant role in the disease process, and the perception of stress is amplified in fibromyalgia patients, then we must try to figure out why.

The answer may lie in an individuals' personality.

Many scientists argue that stress response varies individually as it is regulated by a persons' personality[38]. When it comes to fibromyalgia there is no specific personality type that applies to all individuals. However, researchers have noticed common personality traits and behaviours among fibromyalgic patients[38]. It is theorized that these personality traits can heighten a person's stress response which may turn into a negative physical response in the body, leading to fibromyalgia[3].

Having a type-A personality is one of the traits found among fibromyalgia patients that may play a role in increasing disease symptoms[39]. This is a characteristic I can relate to. Since my early academic days of attending a high school for gifted students, I was extremely ambitious, competitive, organized and meticulous with everything I said and did. This extended into my 20s and 30s where I maintained a busy career and robust social life. Another fibromyalgic personality trait researchers have found is perfectionism[40]. I was always aggressively busy, never accepting anything but perfection from myself. I had very little patience for errors or wasted time in my daily schedule. I rarely ever took time to relax in my daily push towards "excellence". When I wasn't working or spending time with friends or family, I was cleaning my house or working out at the gym. Ironically, looking back, I thought I was thriving off my fast-paced lifestyle. This was proved wrong by a study conducted on over 120 female nurses; where it was found that perfectionism inclined a person towards fatigue over time[41].

One medical journal article noted findings of an elevated depression level among fibromyalgia patients who exhibited difficulty relaxing; trouble sharing feelings and emotions with others and a decreased desire to socialize[42]. Another study had similar findings, where a pessimistic personality type that constantly worries about the future was linked to fibromyalgia sufferers[43].

When a human is faced with a stressor they must utilize coping mechanisms, which are a key to survival and positive progression in life. Unfortunately, these coping mechanisms towards stress and pain in patients with fibromyalgia syndrome are different from those who are healthy[44]. When you think about it, our reactions towards stress are a means of survival. For example, when a person is under a lot of pressure they may suddenly feel their heart race, begin sweating and feel tingly in the arms and legs. We call this anxiety and when even more intense, it is labelled as panic. Our body is getting ready for combat (fight) or running away (flight) as a way of protection. Sometimes there is also dizziness and poor thought processing as blood rushes away from the brain to the extremities (arms and legs) to assist with the protective response of fighting. This is normal! Anxiety can be viewed here as a normal bodily response! Well, in most cases. Fibromyalgia patients seem to have trouble using positive coping mechanisms; whereas healthy individuals may be able to change their emotional experience of pain to one that is less terrible, by using positive thinking.

Women with fibromyalgia often use avoidance and have a higher level of anger as an emotional response, when compared to other healthy females[45]. So what does this all mean? Was I a 'Debbie Downer' all those years ago? Was my temperament causing my own pain and inability to cope with stress? Were my subconscious, negative, thought cycles which hyper-focused on perfectionism and my future, making me a target for this stress-related illness?

The real, honest answer is: Perhaps.

We as humans have the capability to change our perceptions of stress and regulate how we respond to it. My poor responses to stress after my car accident may have played a large part in prolonging my fibromyalgia symptoms. This was a vicious cycle where my negative emotional responses to stress made my physical fibromyalgia pain worst.

It is vital to note that none of this is the fault of the fibromyalgia sufferer. Remember those stressful life events we discussed before? Well, these unavoidable stressful life events combined with the fact that we may hold some character traits which make us susceptible to falling victim to our experiential traumas, are a recipe for disaster. This is not in the conscious control of a fibromyalgic individual.

In the end, we need to emphasize throughout this discussion that beyond all the stress and personality quirks, there is a neurochemical imbalance here. Mainly with the neurotransmitters serotonin, dopamine and norepinephrine as discussed earlier. These chemical imbalances in the body will affect our sleep, energy, motivation, pain modulation pathways, behaviour and even our response to stress[46].

So, how can we as fibromyalgia patients begin to build resiliency to the stressors in our lives? Beyond bringing awareness to our thoughts and responses, the answer to this question may be linked to balancing our stress hormone, cortisol.

THE CORTISOL CONNECTION

Cortisol is the stress hormone made in our body via two organs. The adrenal glands that produce cortisol can be found above each of your kidneys. Cortisol is known for its role in the body's "fight or flight" response. This is when we experience a stressor and regions in our brain known as the pituitary gland and hypothalamus, signal the adrenals to make cortisol and adrenaline. The resultant increased blood levels of stress hormone put the body on high alert. This then assists the body in defending or fleeing the stressor. Cortisol does this by shutting off or slowing down some body functions. By temporarily taking energy away from the reproductive system, immunity, growth and digestion for example, cortisol allows the body to use more of its energy to focus on fighting or fleeing the crisis/threat. There are cortisol receptors all over the body to make this possible. Cortisol even increases blood sugar (glucose) levels to assist with the increased energy needs during the stress response. Adrenaline on the other hand increases heart rate. This gets blood to the arms and legs fast, in preparation to run or fight amidst the stress.

Cortisol also plays a role in human motivation, learning and memory. It regulates our sleep and wake cycle. It plays a role in decreasing inflammation. Cortisol regulates blood pressure and even how the body processes fats, protein and carbohydrates from food. That's why stress hormone is so greatly implicated in fibromyalgia brain fog, insomnia and weight gain.

At this point, you may be thinking cortisol seems great. It helps protect us from danger, and even boosts our energy when we need it. Also, once the stressor or threat is gone, cortisol will help the body readjust to a normal functioning.

However, the problems begin when cortisol levels become imbalanced. Too high when they should be low and too low when they should be high. Some integrative doctors refer to this as "adrenal fatigue".

One way cortisol could become too high is via a tumor growing on the adrenal glands which can cause excess cortisol production. More commonly though an out of whack cortisol level is due to prolonged excessive stress; where the fight or flight response stays "on" instead of shutting off and returning the body to its healthy pre-stress condition[47]. This irregular fluctuation of stress hormone can negatively affect our stress response. This cortisol imbalance is linked to sleep disorders, decreased pain tolerance, heart disease, anxiety/depression, poor digestion, increased weight and even chronic headaches[47].

Higher cortisol levels have been linked to depression[48], whereas lower levels are associated with post traumatic stress disorder[49]. A recent study found that high levels of cortisol in the body can even have an impact on genetic and DNA processes[50]. The American Sleep Disorders Association found a link between sleep loss and higher cortisol fluctuations[51].

It is clear that regulating the stress hormone can help some fibromyalgic individuals. Later in this book I will provide some protocols for balancing

cortisol and supporting the adrenal glands.

DIET MATTERS

Do you ever notice being completely exhausted and feeling lethargic by mid-afternoon? I'm talking about falling asleep at your desk at work; having difficulty concentrating and "needing" a coffee; or worse, having intense cravings for sugar during this low energy period. This energy low is linked to a stress hormone (cortisol) imbalance. As a result, this imbalance increases our body's demand for energy which causes that "I need sugar or coffee now or I am going to pass out at my desk" feeling. In response to this, you may grab a mid-afternoon snack. Let's say a coffee and a muffin; maybe some fast-food; potato chips and soda; or fruit and yogurt. Well, science has shown us that during stressful times, the foods we choose to eat are often high in fat or sugar content[52]. Our mood and stress-levels can have a large impact on what we eat. Humans will often turn to high calorie comfort foods, even when they don't feel hungry or need the calories[53]. This puts us at a disadvantage because what we eat matters!

Remember that our stress hormone, cortisol also plays a role in how we metabolize food (fats, carbohydrates and protein). So, as we are eating our high fat and high sugar foods to boost our low mood and low energy mid-afternoon, we are actually spiking our blood sugar levels. Once the cells in our body are done taking up the sugar we've ingested the leftover amounts of sugar get stored and turned to fat. This fat loves to collect in a few key places-our upper arms, abdominal area/waist, as well as our thighs. This may also be where many fibromyalgia patients and people in general find it the hardest to shed weight. The abdominal adiposity was an area of great frustration for me over the past years. I had a huge gut.

A better alternative mid-afternoon snack would be a high protein, low sugar and even healthy fat snack. Avoiding a sugar spike will better stabilize the blood sugar and insulin levels in the body. This is a key feature of a proper fibromyalgia diet. An example of this would be: a cup of homemade lentil soup, some raw almond butter with low sugar fruit such as an apple, an avocado on a rice cracker, a piece of lean, grilled chicken breast and even an assortment of raw, crunchy vegetables. All these choices are better than fried, processed and refined sugary snacks.

Also, the high fat and high sugar foods we often gravitate towards are full of animal proteins which contain molecules called arachidonic acid. These molecules can increase inflammation in the body. Similarly, animal products we eat can increase our own production of pro-inflammatory molecules called prostaglandins in the body, which have been linked to fibromyalgia pain.

In the United States, the Dietary Guidelines Advisory Committee in a report for the Washington Office of Disease Prevention and Health Promotion recommended following a diet focused on plant-based foods rich in nuts, seeds, vegetables, beans, legumes and whole grains[54].

If you have fibromyalgia, but don't think you can commit to a strict plant based diet there are more practical options. A better approach for many is a diet composed of lean meats (mainly chicken and fish), fruits, vegetables, legumes and minimal amounts of simple carbohydrates (this includes white bread and white rice, cakes, pasta, cookies, donuts etc).

To simplify, we need to cut out the refined carbohydrates for a two main reasons. First, items like white bread, white rice and pasta have very little beneficial fibre and spike our blood sugar. Secondary to this, eliminating sugar via simple carbohydrates (i.e. cakes, muffins, cookies and donuts) may decrease the chances that yeast living in our body will overgrow as they also feed on the sugar that we eat.

One type of this yeast is Candida albicans. Candida has been found in our guts. When Candida overgrows by being in an environment (our body) with lots of available food (high blood sugar) it can aggravate inflammation, allergies, autoimmune disease and may even aggravate the pain of fibromyalgia[55]. So controlling our sugar intake will limit our yeast overgrowth. Furthermore, yeast overgrowth has been linked to an exacerbation of muscle and joint pain[56]. This could be demonstrated by someone suffering from arthritis that may be making their joint pain worst by simply eating too much sugar and causing too much yeast to overgrow.

It is important to note, if you are fibromyalgic and tested positive for celiac disease or gluten sensitivity then you must avoid all grains/gluten containing foods. For those individuals that have not heard of this condition, gluten is basically a bunch of different proteins found in grains such as wheat, barley, rye, and some oats. Individuals will be either very allergic or mildly sensitive to these proteins. In celiac disease the body has an abnormal immune reaction to the wheat proteins, wreaking havoc on digestion. The consumption of gluten in cereal, bread, pasta etc can trigger inflammation in a person who is gluten sensitive for days to months. This may also aggravate the fatigue associated with fibromyalgia.

Higher trace amounts of heavy metals such as lead, cadmium and nickel have also been found in patients with inflammatory conditions[57]. Hence, it is also important for the fibromyalgia patient to try to eat organic foods and consume filtered water as a method of avoiding pesticides, heavy metals and other unhealthy contaminants.

When it comes to my beverage of choice, there were days before my fibromyalgia remission where I was consuming 6 cups of coffee at work. Since then, I always suggest my patients attempt to limit their coffee intake to 1 small cup per day or 2 cups of decaf. Stimulants like caffeine found in coffee, tea and colas do provide short term energy. Unfortunately, these stimulants also make our fatigue worst long-term. The fake boost of energy provided is often followed by sedation (sleepy, drowsy and anxious feelings) which can turn into chronic fatigue. I once had a patient report back to me that cutting out caffeine brought her fibromyalgia pain down to fifty percent. Three months later she went into full remission once we started supplements, swimming daily at her local YMCA and an acupuncture protocol. This exemplifies again that what we consume matters!

So, how does food intake specifically affect pain during a fibromyalgia flare-up? One way of answering this question is by looking at the NMDA (N-methyl-D-aspartate) pain receptors in the body. These NMDA receptors are glutamate receptors, activated when the neurotransmitter glutamate binds to them. So when NMDA pain receptors are bound by glutamate, they get excited and create signal pathways in the brain that have been linked to chronic pain[58].

Fibromyalgic patients have been found to have an increased amount of NMDA receptors as well as overly active NMDA pain receptors[59]. Avoiding dietary sources of substances that mess with these receptors may be a key in reducing a frequency of chronic body pain, headaches and fibromyalgic pain sensitivity. Excitotoxins are substances found in our food that can over stimulate these NMDA pain receptors. An example of this is monosodium glutamate (MSG) and nitrates found in processed foods. These additives can be found in ham, bacon, sauces, potato chips, soups and really almost any other prepared food. MSG and nitrates are often used to preserve and enhance taste. The free glutamate in these foods will cause a glutamate spike in the bloodstream and result in an eventual overstimulation of the NMDA receptors. When experimenting with fibromyalgia patient diets, one rheumatology study found the dietary excitotoxins MSG and aspartame created a worsening of body pain and irritable bowel syndrome among fibromyalgic subjects[60].

As aspartame may also act on the NMDA receptors, I have avoided it as part of my fibromyalgia protocol. I understand how difficult it is to cut synthesized, yet low calorie sweeteners like aspartame from our diet. I used to love diet soda! However, the calorie-free sweetness is not worth the potential headaches and pain for those of us who are sensitive to aspartame[61].

My Fibromyalgia patients often ask me if they should eliminate dairy. Is dairy really bad for us?

A lot of Naturopathic Doctors will ask you to eliminate milk, cheese and sometimes eggs completely. However, I generally stick to the Harvard Medical School of Public Health guidelines, where it is recommended to limit dairy products to one or two servings a day[62]. Harvard made this newer guideline because new research has shown that dairy may not be the best source of calcium and may increase the risks of some types of cancers[62]. An alternative approach would be to consume dark leafy greens such as kale, collard greens, broccoli and bok choy etc. These are rich in calcium too.

Many experts believe that drinking milk from animals may also progress the pain symptoms of fibromyalgia in humans. This has been a passionately debated topic and is still under scientific investigation. However, one medical hypothesis states that the saturated fat and allergens in cows' milk may be the major trigger for developing chronic inflammatory disorders[63]. Ultimately, inflammation equals pain, so it is best to limit consumption of dairy as Harvard has suggested. Again, it is important to note that some individuals may be more sensitive to dairy than others.

A similar dietary challenge for us fibromyalgic individuals is whether or not we should eat nightshades. Nightshades are plants we consume from the Solanaceae family. These include foods like potatoes, peppers, tomatoes, zucchini and eggplant. These plants contain substances called alkaloids in them. They may be pro-inflammatory in some particularly sensitive individuals. A few patients with fibromyalgia, chronic fatigue syndrome and rheumatoid arthritis within my private practice have eliminated these foods and noticed a decrease in joint and muscle pain. Other patients have noticed no notable change. Currently, there is no solid scientific evidence to prove that nightshades cause inflammation in the people that consume them. In fact, most research focuses on the antioxidant and vitamin content of peppers and tomatoes, promoting their consumption. As a solution, it may be advantageous to eliminate these foods for 3 weeks from your diet then slowly incorporate them back in. This may help to decipher if there are any negative or positive reactions.

Our fibromyalgia diet protocol will be richer in cruciferous vegetables such as broccoli, cabbage, cauliflower, kale, Brussels sprouts and asparagus; as these super foods support the liver and assist in balancing hormones. Please refer to the Fibromyalgia Diet Protocol in this book for a more comprehensive fibromyalgia dietary guideline and sample meal plans.

SEDENTARY TO SICK

Once you get your hormones, pain, diet and stress under control, the next phase of reaching fibromyalgia remission is to start moving!

I understand you are in pain. Exercise may be the last thing you want to do. When I was at the worst point of my own fibromyalgic pain I stopped exercising. I physically could not execute my morning run anymore. In retrospect, stopping all cardio and never trying to find an alternative exercise I was comfortable with, wasn't the smartest decision. This caused my muscles to get weak. They got so weak that at one point I had difficulty climbing the stairs and getting in and out of the bathtub. A recent study concluded that women with fibromyalgia were less physically active and spent more time being sedentary (sitting) than healthy women who were the same age[64].

Could the lack of exercise and movement be contributing to pain and stiffness experienced with fibromyalgia? It does seem like a vicious cycle where the pain stops us from exercising and the exercising aggravates the fibromyalgia pain.

Research has actually shown that aggressive exercise can make fibromyalgia symptoms worst in patients[65]. The solution to this is to limit one's exercise to what one can tolerate and to avoid vigorous physical activity; while also avoiding becoming sedentary and inactive. This can be done via low-intensity cardiovascular endurance training[66].

One study found that experiences of widespread muscle pain and tender points reportedly decreased in fibromyalgia subjects after they engaged in aerobic endurance exercise[67]. These patients were put on an exercise schedule where they jogged, walked, cycled or went swimming for 12 weeks[67]. Swimming and water aerobics in particular have been beneficial to many of my fibromyalgia patients. Research has shown that similar to walking; swimming can reduce pain and stiffness among fibromyalgic individuals as well as increase their overall physical functioning[68]. Water therapy is great because there is no gravity and the body often feels light and easier to move. However, the cardiovascular endurance exercise of swimming laps, wading or even completing an aerobics class in the pool should also be done to tolerance.

Another potentially advantageous exercise for fibromyalgia patients is resistant exercises. These exercises could include light free weights (dumbbells or kettlebells) or even light resistant bands. Some gyms also have resistant cables, which allow you to move your arms or legs while applying resistance through a hydraulic band attached to a machine. Over time the weight or resistance can be increased to tolerance. Researchers found that resistance exercises have been shown to increase muscle tone,

and also improve physical fatigue in fibromyalgia patients[69]. These findings were true for women who completed resistant

exercises twice a week for 15 weeks[69].

The above findings really emphasize how important physical fitness is when it comes to pain and the overall vitality of fibromyalgia sufferers. We will discuss a fibromyalgia exercise plan later on in this book.

DIFFERENTIAL DIAGNOSIS

How is Fibromyalgia Diagnosed?

The American College of Rheumatology recently created new criteria to assist with diagnosing fibromyalgia[70]. These parameters use a scale to assess widespread pain on the right and left side of the body, as well as above and below the waist. Another scale is used to assess how intense and bad your symptoms actually are. A diagnosis of fibromyalgia is based on the following factors:

1. You have a widespread pain index measurement score at a level of seven or higher and a symptom severity scale score of five or higher[70].

2. You may also present with a widespread pain index measurement score at a level of three to six and a symptom severity scale of nine or higher[70].

3. You have experienced these symptoms consistently for three months or longer[70].

4. There are no other disorders or illnesses that you may have which could explain your fibromyalgia symptoms[70].

This new system for testing fibromyalgic patients who present with widespread pain is much better than the older system. The older system had doctors simply apply pressure to eighteen designated tender points on the body and see if eleven or more of these points caused pain.

As we discussed at the beginning of this book, fibromyalgia can look like many other health disorders because of the wide range of symptoms a patient may experience. Subsequently, I always recommend that my patients keep a health diary, where they can write down daily struggles with symptoms to share with their health care practitioner. This can speed up diagnosis and treatment. There are also various types of blood work that one can get to help differentiate fibromyalgia syndrome from other causes of pain and illness.

LAB TESTS FOR THE FIBROMYALGIA PATIENT

Complete Blood Count (CBC)

A complete blood count test will measure your red blood cell, white blood cell and platelet levels via a small blood sample taken from the vein. Of particular interest is MCV (Mean Corpuscular Volume) and MCH (Mean Corpuscular Hemoglobin).

The MCV blood test is a measurement of the average red blood cell size. When this measurement shows up to be abnormally high on your blood work it may indicate a vitamin B12 and/or folic acid deficiency. This is known as macrocytic anemia. When the MCV blood test levels are abnormally low on your blood work, this may indicate an iron deficiency in the body. This is known as microcytic anemia. Anemia can cause patients to complain of low energy, extreme fatigue, increased heart beat, dizziness, difficulty concentrating, headache and even insomnia. It is easy to see why a CBC test is important; as symptoms of anemia are very similar to some major fibromyalgic complaints. Hence, it is important to rule out vitamin and nutrient deficiencies as a contributing factor here.

The MCH blood test is a measurement of the average hemoglobin amount in our red blood cells. Hemoglobin is a protein found in all red blood cells. It is a carrier of oxygen which the red blood cells deliver from the lungs to the body. MCH levels can be abnormally low or high on blood work when there is anemia caused by malnutrition. A high MCH on blood work may also indicate infection, cancer complications, overactive thyroid gland and liver disease[71].

Thyroid Function Tests

Earlier we discussed the low metabolism theory of fibromyalgia and its connection to the thyroid. Scientists approximate that around 90% of fibromyalgia patients have some level of thyroid dysfunction[17]. It is important to check thyroid hormone levels via a TSH, T3 and T4 blood test to rule out any problems with thyroid functioning.

A TSH (Thyroid Stimulating Hormone) blood test will measure how much thyroid stimulating hormone is in your blood. The TSH is produced in the brain by the pituitary gland. When our TSH levels are abnormally high in the body; it can indicate low thyroid functioning or hypothyroidism. In this case the brain is producing more and more TSH to signal the thyroid gland to produce more T3 and T4 thyroid hormones because is not producing enough.

When the TSH is abnormally low, the thyroid may be overactive and produce too much T3 and T4. TSH levels would drop here; as the body does not want to stimulate the thyroid to make any more hormones. This is known as hyperthyroidism.

A T4 (thyroxine) thyroid hormone test will check how much T4 is being produced by your thyroid gland. A T3 (triiodothyronine) blood test will measure the blood levels of the more active thyroid hormone, T3. As both T3 and T4 thyroid hormones are produced directly by the thyroid gland, any abnormal increases or decreases in their levels may indicate a thyroid disorder.

Thyroid Autoimmune Markers

So let's say that your thyroid hormone levels come back abnormal on your blood work report. Your doctor may suspect that you have a thyroid autoimmune disease. This is when our immune system creates cells called antibodies which wrongly attack our own thyroid gland and various thyroid proteins. This can cause improper thyroid functioning and a poor production of T3 and T4. Hence, a fibromyalgia patient may not just have hypothyroidism. They may have hypothyroidism due to an autoimmune disorder.

Hashimoto's Thyroiditis is an autoimmune disease that causes hypothyroidism. Many fibromyalgia symptoms, such as fatigue, dry skin, weight gain and depression can mimic the symptoms of Hashimoto's disease. Additionally, research has found that many Hashimoto's sufferers also have fibromyalgia syndrome[72]. This exemplifies the importance of investigating autoimmune thyroid disorders that can not only mimic fibromyalgia but also occur alongside it.

Thyroid Peroxidase Antibody (TPOAb) blood testing will detect such an autoimmune disease. TPO (thyroid peroxidase) is an enzyme which can be found in the thyroid gland. It plays a role in converting a storage protein called thyroglobulin into T3 and T4 hormones. TPO Antibody will obstruct T3 and T4 production by attacking the TPO enzyme; resulting in hypothyroid functioning.

Another blood test to consider is Thyroglobulin Antibody (TGAb). Remember, the thyroid hormones T3 and T4 are produced from the protein thyroglobulin which is stored in the thyroid. The thyroglobulin antibodies can target the thyroglobulin protein, causing inflammation and damage to the thyroid gland, while also creating low functioning.

If your thyroid is hyperactive and your blood work comes back with a low TSH and high T3, T4 blood levels, then your doctor might suspect Grave's Disease. This is not a common scenario among most fibromyalgia patients. However, I wanted to add in that a TSHRAb (Thyroid Stimulating Hormone Receptor Antibody) test can be done. This blood test will look for antibodies which affect the receptors on the thyroid where thyroid stimulating hormone (TSH) would normally bind. These antibodies stimulate these TSH receptors and cause the thyroid to grow. As a result, this enlargement also creates more and more T3 and T4 thyroid hormone production or hyperthyroidism.

Rheumatoid Factor

Rheumatoid Factor (RF) is another autoimmune protein that is produced by the body. Rheumatoid Factor can target healthy tissue and joints causing pain and inflammation. A diagnosis of rheumatoid arthritis (RA) is confirmed when RF is found to be high on blood tests.

There are various clinical cases where patients with RA have been misdiagnosed as having fibromyalgia due to the many shared symptoms[73]. Hence, Rheumatoid Factor blood testing will help clearly differentiate the diseases.

Cyclic Citrullinated Peptide Test (optional)

A cyclic citrullinated peptide antibody test is another marker of rheumatoid arthritis that can be tested for via blood work. This test will also give insight into the severity of the rheumatoid arthritis.

ESR

Erythrocyte Sedimentation Rate (ESR) is a blood test which uses red blood cell patterns, to confirm the presence of inflammation. Although this test will tell us if there is inflammation in the body, it does not specifically tell us where the inflammation is occurring. It is still a helpful blood test to have.

CRP

C - reactive protein (CRP) is a protein produced in the liver in response to inflammation. Blood tests that show CRP levels above normal indicate some inflammatory trauma in the body. Researchers have reported finding a higher level of CRP among fibromyalgia patients; especially overweight fibromyalgic individuals[74]. This test may assist us in deciphering whether or not our body pain and joint stiffness symptoms are related to inflammation.

Stool Ova Parasite Test

Many fibromyalgia patients will present with gastrointestinal complaints. These symptoms may include alternating stools (where our bowel movements will switch between consti-pation and diarrhea); abdominal cramping; bloating; gas and pain. The occurrence of irritable bowel syndrome (IBS) has been found to be higher in fibromyalgia patients than in non-fibromyalgia patients[75]. So why is fibromyalgia associated with a 1.5 times increased risk for IBS?[76] There is no conclusive scientific evidence to answer this question. Some medical prac-titioners believe that IBS may occur similarly, and often along side with fibromyalgia[75]. For example, IBS presents with an in-creased pain sensitivity which may involve dysfunctional anti-nociceptive pathways (pain-blocking nerve pathways) and ab-normal serotonin levels in the body[76]. As discussed in the last chapter, these are all potential causal factors for fibromyalgia. IBS has also been reported to be brought on by emotional and physical stressors.

A recent study found that patients with IBS have a greater pres-ence of parasites in their digestive tract, compared to people without IBS[77]. Researchers who conducted this study believe that the parasites found in IBS patients, which include Giardia, Cryptosporidium and even Blastocystis, may play a role in the actual disease process[77]. When it comes to the fibromyalgic sufferer, it is important to rule out parasites as a cause for the irregular bowl movements and the digestive pain/discomfort. An ova and parasite test can identify parasitic eggs and grown parasites in the body. This test is done by collecting a small stool sample which is then sent to the lab for testing. This test will assist your doctor in determining if he or she should pre-scribe any antibiotic or antiparasitic medication such as Metro-nidazole to you.

Within my clinical practice, we generally provide each patient with a series of three ova and parasite testing kits to avoid miss-ing any undetected parasites in their poo. The ova and parasite testing kit consists of a tube which contains preserving liquid and a small collection scoop attached to a lid. Now before you get uncomfortable, rest assured you can take this kit home to prepare the sample before returning it to a clinic or lab. An easy way to take this test is to have a bowel movement in a plastic bag, or on a piece of saran wrap covering the toilet. We do not want water, urine or any other contaminants touching the fecal sample. A few scoops of the stool can then be taken using the kit. When taking these samples try to collect bloody, discoloured or slimy sections. For difficult and dry stools taking samples from the center of the bowel movement will suffice. The stool ova and parasite test has demystified the cause of digestive complaints and even food sensitivities among many of my fibromyalgia patients.

Celiac Testing

As discussed earlier, Celiac disease is an autoimmune disorder where your own immune system will react negatively to the gluten that you have eaten. This causes the intestines to become inflamed, sensitive and even damaged. Not only can this cause extreme abdominal pain and digestive upset, it can also interfere with our ability to absorb vitamins and nutrients in the gut. Ultimately, this can lead to extreme fatigue, weak bones, infertility, and in rare cases cancer. There are also many patients who do not have autoimmune celiac disease but still feel unwell when they eat gluten. We will refer to these patients as non-celiac gluten sensitive (NCGS).

Gluten, as you already know is a protein found in various grains. Celiac patients may react to the protein Gliadin that is found in wheat; the protein Secalin found in Rye; the protein Hordein in Barley; and less commonly the protein Avenin in Oats.
Wheat sensitive patients may also react to wheat derived substances such as bulgar, semolina, faro, kamut etc. (as they also contain gluten). Unfortunately, celiac patients can also react to gluten-free corn and rice based cereals and pastas, simply because these foods have come in contact with a gluten containing grain through factory processing. The cross-contamin-

ation of food with gluten is a major source of frustration for many people. Recently, food manufacturers in North America have begun to specify if a product is gluten free and free from contamination.

Within my private practice I was shocked to find some individuals to be so intensely sensitive to gluten proteins that even touching the grains could create a reaction. One patient in particular would get itchy bumps on her skin from simply leaning on the kitchen counter and accidently contacting breadcrumbs left behind by a family member. I have also had celiac and NCGS patients report being aggravated by licking a stamp's gluten-containing adhesive; drinking wine that was aged in oak barrels sealed with a paste made of flour; or wearing lipstick and other cosmetic products which contain gluten proteins.

Researchers have found a high occurrence of celiac disease and non-celiac gluten sensitivity (NCGS) among fibromyalgia patients[78]. One European study even listed non-celiac gluten sensitivity as a potential cause of fibromyalgia. This was after extensive experiments' where fibromyalgia patients who were not celiac, found relief from their irritable bowels, muscle pain and low energy once they were placed on a strict gluten-free diet[79].

To test for Celiac disease, an intestinal biopsy may also be ordered by your doctor. Most physicians believe this is the gold standard and the most reliable test to confirm a celiac diagnosis. During this procedure a tiny piece of your small intestine will be removed and sent to a lab for analysis. Due to this being mildly invasive, many patients will opt to receive the following blood work first:

Tissue Transglutaminase Antibodies Test (tTG-IgA): In celiac disease our immune system reacts with gluten creating antibodies that attack an intestinal enzyme called tissue transglutaminase. A tissue transglutaminase antibody test specifically measures these antibody levels. It can also be used to monitor progress of treatment, as the antibody levels should drop once gluten is no longer entering the body.

<u>Deamidated Gliadin IgG antibodies</u>: A very small percentage of celiac patients have a deficiency of antibodies called IgA[80]. This creates a false negative result of the above tTG-IgA test, as no tissue transglutaminase antibodies are detected in the blood[80]. To counteract this, a Deamidated Gliadin IgG test is often used. This tests for the antibody IgG which may be positive in some celiac patients who tested negatively for tTG-IgA.

<u>IgA Anti-Gliadin Antibodies</u>: These antibodies are created in the body against the wheat protein Gliadin. They are found in approximately 8 out of 10 people with celiac disease[80].

There are also genetic tests available for the celiac disease markers known as HLA DQ2 and HLA DQ8.

It is important to note that the blood tests to rule out celiac disease should be performed while you are still consuming gluten in your diet and subsequently, producing antibodies in reaction.

<u>Non-celiac Gluten Sensitivity (NCGS) Testing</u>
People suffering from NCGS lack the autoimmune markers that celiac disease causes. The intestinal lining of an individual with NCGS may still have some mild abnormalities. More significant are the symptoms experienced with this gluten sensitivity. These may include joint pain, headaches, nausea, tiredness, nasal congestion, skin rashes, bloating, mental fatigue and fogginess, abdominal pain and diarrhea or constipation[79].

With no autoimmune markers and a negative biopsy for celiac disease, how do we diagnose this gluten sensitivity in non-celiac patients?

After receiving a negative celiac test, the best way to determine if you are gluten sensitive or intolerant is to completely cut out gluten from your diet. This gluten elimination diet should last for at least one month. There are many resources available which cover what to eat during a gluten-free diet. Once the diet has commenced you can assess how you feel without gluten.

After about 4 weeks on the gluten-free diet, you can eat some gluten containing food. At this point you will need to monitor your body and any symptoms that arise for four days after eating gluten again. If you notice your fibromyalgia or IBS symptoms flaring up with gluten intake, it can indicate sensitivity and a need for dietary changes. Later, we will discuss some alternative treatment options to increase the health of the gut and decrease food sensitivities among fibromyalgia patients.

Nerve conduction Test
Fibromyalgia patients may report experiencing weird sensations like coldness, burning, sharp and tingling pain in various parts of their body. I often struggled with burning and electric shock like sensations in my neck and upper back. Some days I also had a feeling of pins-and-needles which turned to numbness in my right hand. Your doctor may diagnose this as peripheral neuropathy. This basically means that there is damage to the nerves that exist outside the central nervous system (brain and spinal cord). When it comes to nerve pain in the body, it is not surprising to learn that almost fifty percent of fibromyalgia syndrome patients' have some damage to their peripheral small nerve fibers[81]. A nerve conduction test known as electromyography (EMG) can check the health of our muscles and nerves and assist in diagnosing this peripheral nerve damage[82].

Nerves communicate information to other nerves in the body via electric signals they generate. To perform an EMG, your doctor will insert a needle into a muscle. An electric pulse will then travel through this needle to the nerves in the muscle. The resulting electrical activity is then recorded. During an EMG test, your doctor may also apply electrode stickers to your muscles and measure how strong and how fast electricity moves from one muscle point to another. The EMG patterns of some fibromyalgia patients have shown slower electrical signalling[83].

Punch Biopsy

Some physicians prefer an in-office procedure called a skin punch biopsy. This is where they cut a small section of the patient's skin to test under a microscope for nerve damage. This skin punch biopsy has been said to be easier and a lot less painful than EMG nerve conduction tests[84].

Many neurologists claim that individuals who present with chronic and excessive pain which they describe as stabbing, burning and tingling may actually be experiencing the degeneration of small nerves in the body[84]. This may mimic or overlap fibromyalgia and should be assessed, diagnosed and treated separately[83].

Hormone Panel

A complete blood hormone panel will include the following steroid hormones: estradiol (an estrogen), progesterone, luteinizing hormone (LH), follicle stimulating hormone (FSH) and dehydroepiandrosterone (DHEA). Some doctors will also run a free testosterone test to check for infertility in men and to rule out polycystic ovarian syndrome in women.

A recent study examined women with migraines who also suffered from a decreased production of these steroid hormones[85]. This group of women were especially deficient in progesterone production[85]. They were treated with hormone restorative therapy via the use of bioidentical hormones[85]. These hormones are made in a lab by various pharmaceutical companies, but they are identical to the hormones produced by the body. The researchers concluded that the hormonal imbalance these women had was the cause of their migraines. This was exemplified after the bioidentical hormone replacement caused their migraines, insomnia, depression, digestive complaints and fibromyalgia to disappear[85].

Over the many years in my private practice, the number one complaint I have received from women who are entering menopause is insomnia. This is often described as difficulty falling asleep at night. It would take some of my patients anywhere from thirty minutes to 3 hours to initiate sleep. If you are a fibromyalgic woman above the age of 40 and you experience insomnia, hot flashes and irregular periods, this may be due to perimenopausal hormonal imbalance. A hormone blood test can shed light on this.

Studies in sleep disorders have also found that the higher levels of substance P and lower levels of serotonin among fibromyalgia patients can affect mood and sleep significantly[86]. It is important to rule out hormonal imbalance that could be making these fibromyalgia symptoms worst.

Some women with fibromyalgia do not have abnormal hormone levels. However, a few long term studies have shown that even normal daily fluctuations of progesterone and testosterone may be associated with how intensely a fibromyalgic woman will experience pain[87].

<u>Cortisol Testing</u>

Earlier we discussed the stress hormone cortisol and its role in the fibromyalgia stress response. There are various ways to check cortisol levels in the body if your doctor suspects an imbalance. These include cortisol testing through saliva, urine or blood. A salivary cortisol test is quite easy to do as it only requires collecting saliva at various times throughout the day to send to a lab for analysis. We need to be mindful that some patients may find collecting their urine or giving blood samples to be stressful. This stress response will naturally increase cortisol production and may elevate test results.

When assessing fibromyalgia patients, cortisol was found to be lower in patients who experienced greater fatigue and sleep disturbances[88]. Cortisol levels were also linked to the number of tender points these patients experienced[88]. Some researchers believe that low morning cortisol levels can contribute to depression among fibromyalgic patients[89].

An alternative medicine view of chronic stress causing chronic fatigue is referred to as adrenal fatigue or hypoandrenia. This is when a person is under constant stress causing the adrenal glands to produce high amounts of the stress hormone cortisol in response. Eventually, this individual will become so fatigued and cannot produce consistent amounts of cortisol anymore. The result is a cortisol (stress hormone) imbalance in the body. Although many doctors' use this as a diagnosis, there is actually no concrete research to validate "adrenal fatigue" as a medical condition. In fact, a recent study on endocrine disorders deemed it as non-existent[90]. This is a huge area of debate among many physicians from all fields of practice.

Regardless, the symptoms of fatigue, sugar cravings, anxiety and depression, insomnia and weight gain are real. Subsequently, how can we approach a fluctuating and imbalanced cortisol level? Why can't we just replace the cortisol when it becomes too low? Well, cortisol replacement (even tiny doses) is very dangerous and can cause many side-effects like diabetes, cardiovascular disease and weight gain. Luckily, cortisol testing can provide some insight into hormonal imbalance. This can then be addressed through stress management, lifestyle, nutritional and supplement interventions which are tailored to the fibromyalgic individual.

Blood Sugar Testing

Two blood tests I regularly run on my fibromyalgia patients are a Fasting Glucose Test and a Hemoglobin A1C test. The fasting glucose test is performed after the patient has not eaten overnight for 8-10 hours. This test tells us how much sugar is in the patients' blood stream on the day of the blood draw. Diabetic patients will still show elevated blood sugar levels, despite fasting. The Hemoglobin A1C test on the other hand, will allow us to measure the average blood sugar in the body over the past two to three months. This test is excellent at monitoring diabetes progress. A high A1C will show that an individual is not controlling their blood sugar well.

A paper published in *Rheumatology International* noted

fibromyalgia to be a familiar diagnosis among diabetes patients[91]. These patients also reported experiencing a greater level of pain and had higher hemoglobin A1C levels[91]. Researchers noted that the fibromyalgia syndrome may be a complication of the diabetes which could be regulated by simply normalizing the blood sugar level[91].

<u>Sleep Apnea Testing</u>
Many years ago, scientists found sleep apnea occurring among a large portion of male fibromyalgia syndrome patients[92]. Sleep apnea is a disorder where your breathing can pause for up to thirty seconds during sleep. This can occur numerous times in one night. It is caused by the airway getting blocked by soft or fatty tissue at the back of the throat; a large tongue; a narrow airway or even relaxed throat muscles. During this sleep disturbance a person may begin to loudly snore after a breathing pause or even gasp for breath. Sleep apnea is bad because when we are not breathing our body is not getting enough oxygen. This can create quite a range of negative symptoms, including headaches; fatigue and sleepiness during the day; poor memory and concentration; as well as irritability. One fibromyalgia study found that 50% of females suffering from sleep apnea had chronic pain[93]. These patients who experienced upper airway resistance during sleep also tested positive for fibromyalgia tender points. Despite these findings, there is still much research needed for us to fully understand how the sleep disturbances experienced in fibromyalgia syndrome relate to our depression and pain.

For those patients who have sleep apnea and fibromyalgia a continuous positive airway pressure (CPAP) machine may be prescribed by their doctor. Fibromyalgia patients with sleep apnea who used the CPAP machine at night were found to stay asleep longer and feel less depressed during the day[94]. A sleep apnea test is sometimes referred to as a sleep study. It is often conducted over night in a comfortable laboratory room, set up for sleeping. This is because during the test you will be hooked up to lung, brain and heart monitors as you sleep. The sleep study doctors will then monitor your blood oxygen levels and breathing patterns.

Ferritin

As discussed earlier, a CBC test will help us detect microcytic anemia due to iron deficiency. A ferritin blood test can then be done to confirm iron deficiency or conversely iron overload in the body. Ferritin is a protein that stores iron in the tissues of the body. Hence, in iron deficiency anemia the amount of iron storage is low and ferritin can be seen at below normal values.

Researchers in Europe have found that ferritin levels on blood work below a value of 50ng/ml created over six times an increased risk for fibromyalgia syndrome[95]. This makes sense because iron plays a role in the creation of dopamine and serotonin in the body. They believe this low iron may lead to the low serotonin and dopamine levels seen in fibromyalgia syndrome[95].

Now this research alone is not enough to support the theory that iron deficiency causes muscle pain disorders. However, when our muscles lack access to iron and oxygen they produce less energy. Similar to fibromyalgia, iron deficiency can also cause a person to feel dizzy, tired and weak.

Serum B12

Vitamin B12 which is also called cobalamin is one of the eight B vitamins in the body. It is involved in everything from the creation of DNA to the production of nerves in the brain. Many patients experience a B12 deficiency as fatigue, skin numbness or tingling and poor coordination[96]. Researchers have also found that a long term B12 deficiency can actually damage the brain, causing it to shrink in seniors[96]. This can affect mental processing or cognition[96]. MRI studies can show negative changes in the brain due to B12 deficiency[97]. In these severe cases of deficiency, treatment with B12 may only allow for a partial recovery[97]. This is why treating low B12 levels in the body early is important in improving the life of patients[98].

Researchers have found that patients with fibromyalgia syndrome and chronic fatigue syndrome who took B12 injections with folic acid pills experienced pain relief[99]. Earlier we spoke about nerve damage (neuropathy) among Fibromyalgia patients. Well, scientists have also found a connection between vitamin B12 deficiency and peripheral neuropathy[100]. In one study, nerve damage was reduced and prevented among patients who were given B12 supplementation.

A serum vitamin B12 blood test will assist with diagnosing a deficiency. A normal blood value of B12 can range from 200-1000ng/L. When a person has B12 blood levels below 200ng/L they are positively deficient. However, some individuals may show signs of deficiency at B12 levels below 450ng/L. Some doctors suggest a more specific test called the Methylmalonic Acid blood test. Methylmalonic acid levels in the blood increase as the amount of B12 decreases in the body.

Serum Vitamin D Testing
A vitamin D blood test is known as the 25(OH) Vitamin D or 25-hydroxy Vitamin D test. This is one of the most important blood tests to obtain as a fibromyalgia patient if you live in the northern hemisphere. In Canada for example, after summer ends, there is virtually no vitamin D being made in our bodies during the winter months. This leads to nationwide deficiencies.
I once had a medical professor tell me he averaged himself as making 0 to 200 international units (IUs) of vitamin D a day during winter. He noted his family in the Caribbean were making upwards of 60,000IUs per day. The sun provides UVB rays which our skin uses to create vitamin D which is then activated by our liver and kidneys. Vitamin D can also be found in fatty fish like mackerel and salmon; cheese, egg yolks and beef liver. Often, it is added to milk and orange juice you find in grocery stores.

Scientists have long recognized how important vitamin D is to muscle functioning[101]. One of the signs of vitamin D deficiency is chronic muscle pain and weakness[102]. Low vitamin D levels have also been seen in depressed patients[103]. New research in the fields of nutrition and pain, has found low vitamin D status to be a common occurrence among fibromyalgia patients[104]. They do not know why so many fibromyalgia patients present with low vitamin D. Fibromyalgia researchers suspect that vitamin D is involved somehow in the body's pain pathways [104]. An article published in the Korean Journal of pain even suggests vitamin D supplementation as a method of prevention against fibromyalgia development[105]. This suggestion may be warranted as treating vitamin D deficiency may greatly improve the quality of life among fibromyalgic individuals[106]. This is seen in experiments where fibromyalgia patients who were given vitamin D to treat their deficiency, also experienced an improvement in mood, pain (tender points) and energy[107].

Now, if you are one of those individuals who are diligent about protecting your skin from the sun with sunscreen, clothing or staying indoors, this deficiency could be chronic and extend into the summer season. You may also be at risk for vitamin D deficiency if you are elderly, overweight or have darker skin. In this case, supplementation at the daily recommended dose may be prescribed year round. Measuring an exact deficiency level through a blood test will assist your doctor in determining how much oral vitamin D supplementation you need. Because vitamin D is fat soluble, it can be stored in the body for longer periods. This can actually pose a risk for toxic levels to build up. For this reason it is important to know how much to take for your individual needs.

THE PROTOCOL: FINDING YOUR INDIVIDUALIZED PLAN

Although this book majorly focuses on natural evidence based medicine, we must discuss drug therapy first. I would like to preface this conversation with the following statement: There is no shame in taking pharmaceuticals, especially if they help you feel better! I think we live in a very fear-based society where there is a belief that all drugs are bad. I've even heard some alternative medicine doctors say that drugs only act to keep you in a state of sickness. This is far from the truth. Despite the many drug side effects reported with pharmaceutical use, many of these fibromyalgia drugs have been found to be helpful to patients.

In my experience, drug therapy did initially support my pain management. However, it was ultimately non-restorative for me. This is what caused me to seek out effective alternative medicines to halt my fibromyalgia and put it into remission. There are many patients who have different individualized experiences. Some find pharmaceutical drug therapy to be effective at managing their chronic pain, while others rely solely on natural medicine or a combination of pharmaceuticals and neutraceuticals (natural drugs) as treatment.

Regardless of what you choose to incorporate from this book into your own individually created treatment protocol, it is imperative to speak to your Medical or Naturopathic Doctor first. This is important before beginning drug therapy, heading to your local health food store or visiting a natural pharmacy. The main reason for this is due to the fact that some natural drugs and even foods can interact with pharmaceuticals. Secondly, having your doctor monitor changes in tender muscle points, weight, thyroid hormone and liver enzyme levels will enable you to better track your progress.

THE TOP FIBROMYALGIA PHARMACEUTICALS

The United States Food and Drug Administration have approved the following three pharmaceutical drugs for the treatment of Fibromyalgia[108]:

Pregabalin[(S)-3-(aminomethyl)-5-methylhexanoic acid]
This pharmaceutical is best known by its trade name Lyrica[108]. Pregabalin is actually an anti-seizure medication. However, fibromyalgia syndrome patients are often prescribed this drug. Pregabalin helps to decrease muscle and nerve pain as well as anxiety by binding to protein units in the brain tissue[108].

Duloxetine HCL
This pharmaceutical is best known by its trade name Cymbalta. Duloxetine is a selective serotonin and norepinephrine reuptake inhibitor (aka. SNRI) [108]. This means that this drug allows for more serotonin and norepinephrine to remain by nerve sites in the brain by stopping their uptake. Earlier we discussed the importance of these neurotransmitters in our pain pathways. Subsequently, the SNRI Duloxetine assists in decreasing pain and stiffness in the muscles and bones, as well as reducing depression and anxiety[108].

Milnacipran
This pharmaceutical is best known by its trade name Savella. Like Duloxetine, Milnacipran is also a serotonin and norepin-

ephrine reuptake inhibitor (SNRI) [108]. It assists in the management of fibromyalgia pain and depression by restricting the reuptake of serotonin and norepinephrine at a ratio of 1:3[108]. This significant increase in serotonin creates a reduction of symptoms reported by some fibromyalgia patients. This makes me think back to the serotonin deficiency hypotheses we outlined earlier in this book.

Finally, other comparable antidepressant SNRIs which may be prescribed to you for fibromyalgia symptoms include Venlafaxine (trade name: Effexor) and Desvenlafaxine (trade name Pristiq).

THE NATURAL PATH: AN ALTERNATIVE APPROACH.

Thyroid

Okay, so your doctor has diagnosed you with fibromyalgia and found that you are hypothyroid as well. At this point it is beneficial to begin thyroid hormone therapy. It is important to begin this treatment with physiologic doses. A physiologic dose is basically when you are dosed with a hormone, naturally occurring substance or neurotransmitter at an amount your healthy body would normally produce on its own.

Hypothyroid fibromyalgic patients can be given a synthetic T4/T3 hormone dose at a 4:1 ratio[109]. Alternatively, 60mg or 1 grain of desiccated thyroid can also be given and slowly increased by another 60mg each month[109]. For patients who are euthyroid (those who have a proper functioning thyroid gland), 50 to 75 micrograms of T3 can be dosed with weekly increases of 6.25 micrograms[109]. The tricky part here is figuring out the precise best dose for each individual patient. As salivary and blood serum levels are not good indicators; you will need to be monitored by your doctor closely to adjust dosing based on your body's' response to thyroid hormone therapy.
Alternatively, some of you may choose to be put on a manufactured pharmaceutical dose of thyroid hormone. Taking a stand-

ardized hormone therapy of Levothyroxine, such as Synthroid or Levoxyl would allow for less physician monitoring.

It is important to have an electrocardiogram prior to starting any of the above metabolic thyroid hormone therapies. Taking too much thyroid hormone can also affect the heart and any pre-existing cardiac conditions. Also, if your endocrinologist finds that low cortisol is present too, it is beneficial to begin treatment with physiologic doses of cortisol before starting thyroid hormone therapy.

Once beginning thyroid therapy, every fibromyalgia patient should be aware of thyrotoxicosis. Thyrotoxicosis occurs when there is too much thyroid hormone in the body. The symptoms of this may indicate a medical emergency and should not be taken lightly. Individuals experiencing thyrotoxicosis may have a heart rate over 100 beats per minute; excessive sweating and hot flashes; tremors, anxious and agitated mood; weight loss and fatigue with weakness. Go to the hospital or visit your doctor immediately if you feel this may be happening to you. Also, there are many drugs that may disrupt your metabolic functioning and thyroid treatment outcomes. Speak to your doctor if you are taking any Beta blockers, anti-depressants, narcotics and/or muscle relaxants before beginning thyroid hormone therapy.

Alternative Formulas

What about an alternative route for those with fibromyalgia and hypothyroid symptoms? Maybe, like me, you have a slightly elevated TSH but completely normal T3 and T4 thyroid hormone levels on blood work. There are many thyroid herbal supplements that may be effective in giving the thyroid a boost. These can be a great addition to your fibromyalgia protocol.

Many formulas on the market can be purchased at various health food stores and natural pharmacies. The following are some key components to look for when treating hypothyroid fibromyalgia via natural and herbal supplements:

Iodine

Dose: 150 micrograms (mcg)

Iodine is an essential mineral and a key controller in thyroid function. Iodine is needed to create our thyroid hormones. Hence, both T3 and T4 contain iodine in their composition. Your healthcare practitioner may recommend a thyroid herbal formula that contains iodine at a dose of up to 500 micrograms per day (depending on your level of deficiency and thyroid dysfunction). It is important to follow the specific individualized dose prescribed by your Naturopathic or Medical Doctor. Iodine deficiency can cause hypothyroidism and growth of the thyroid gland. However, taking too much iodine can also be very dangerous and cause hypothyroidism and autoimmune problems[110].

Some thyroid alternative health formulas will have iodine listed as an ingredient in the form of potassium iodide. Herbal formulas will use various plants such as algae, seaweed and kelp which are rich in iodine as a source. Two types of iodine rich brown algae often found in high end thyroid herbal formulas include Oarweed (laminararia digitata) and Norwegian Kelp (ascophyllum nodosum).

L-Tyrosine

Dose: 500-2000mg

L-Tyrosine (also known as tyrosine) is an amino acid produced in our body. Tyrosine assists with making thyroid hormones. Tyrosine also plays a role in the creation of the catecholamine neurotransmitters dopamine, norepinephrine and epinephrine. In earlier chapters of this book we discussed how important these all are and the role they may play in the fibromyalgia disease processes.

In our body, iodine combines with tyrosine to create T3 and T4 thyroid hormones. One study linked low amounts of thyroid hormone to low amounts of tyrosine[111]. This makes sense as a lack of tyrosine would halt production of the thyroid hormones and cause metabolism issues.

During stressful periods, our adrenal glands will release more catecholamine neurotransmitters in response. This allows our brains to function normally under pressure. There is actually an area in the middle of the adrenal glands called the adrenal medulla where tyrosine is used to make epinephrine, dopamine and norepinephrine. After a prolonged stress response and an overproduction of these, our catecholamine neurotransmitter stores can become depleted. However, tyrosine supplementation has been found to enhance brain performance in stressful and demanding times by assisting with replenishment of the depleted catecholamine neurotransmitters[112].

L-tyrosine may also help some individuals with depression and irregular mood[113]. This amino acid supplements' mood boosting effect comes down to its role in dopamine production. If you recall dopamine was found to be low among fibromyalgia sufferers. In the body tyrosine turns into dopamine and dopamine in turn influences serotonin levels. The stress relieving and mood/brain-boosting potentials of L-tyrosine are greatly desired among fibromyalgia and hypothyroid patients.

L-tyrosine intake can occur through eating food that is rich in it. This includes cheese, soybeans, beef, lamb, chicken, fish, pork, nuts, seeds, dairy, beans, whole grains and eggs. However, most research showing positive health effects of L-tyrosine is from purified tyrosine supplements at higher doses than food may allow. Most commonly, L-tyrosine is dosed at 500-2000mg one hour prior to exposure to stressful events[114]. Some patients with digestive discomfort may prefer to split their L-tyrosine doses throughout the day. One experiment noted that 2500mg of L-tyrosine taken three times a day for 2 weeks did not cause any side-effects[115]. Most thyroid supplements contain a much lower dose, around 450mg of L-tyrosine.

Coleus forskohlii

Dose: Coleus forskohlii extract (10% forskolin) 250mg

Coleus forskohlii is an Ayurvedic herb that is also found in many high end thyroid herbal supplements. Ayurvedic Medicine is a 6000 year old medicine from India. Coleus forskohlii is used in the treatment of hypothyroidism because it contains an ingredient called forskolin that may increase our production of thyroid hormones[116].

Forskolin may play a role in helping boost the metabolism of fibromyalgia patients by increasing an enzyme in the body called adenylate cyclase[117]. Adenylate cyclase then will produce a messenger molecule in our body called cyclic adenosine mono phosphate (cAMP)

cAMP has been found to play an important role in the functioning of cells, energy production and the regulation of hormone responses. One study found obese men who took 250mg of the Coleus forskohlii extract twice a day for twelve weeks had a lowered fat mass and an increased lean body mass[118].

Ashwagandha (withania somnifera)

Dose: Ashwagandha root (1.5% withanolides)100mg

Ashwagandha has often been prescribed for thyroid problems in traditional Ayurvedic Medicine. Ashwagandha root extract has been found to stimulate thyroid activity and lower elevated cortisol, improving individual stress response[119]. Withanolides are only one of the many active ingredients found in Ashwagandha.

Hypothyroid patients with abnormally elevated TSH levels were given 600mg of Ashwagandha root extract for 8 weeks. When compared to the placebo group (hypothyroid patients whom did not receive Ashwagandha), these patients showed a greater improvement with better levels of T3, T4 and TSH[120].

Bacopa monnieri

Dose: Bacopa monnieri extract (50% bacosides A and b) 300mg
This is another ayurvedic herbal extract. It comes from the water hyssop plant. Bacopa monnieri has been revered for years for its ability to protect the brain from disease while increasing memory and cognitive brain functioning[121].

It is often added to thyroid herbal formulas as it may increase the concentration of T4 thyroid hormone in the body. In fact, animal studies have shown that Bacopa has incredible thyroid stimulating abilities and increases T4 thyroid hormone concentrations by 41% after 15 days of supplementation[122] The active ingredients called bacosides found in Bacopa monnieri extract may benefit fibromyalgia patients beyond boosting their thyroid hormone levels. Recent scientific research has found that Bacopa calms neuropathic (nerve) pain. It does this by reducing hypersensitivity and lowering pain perception[123].

Blue Flag (Iris Versicolor)
Dose: Blue Flag Root 150mg
Blue Flag is a wild iris plant which grows in the marshes of North America. It is an ancient herbal medicine commonly found in alternative thyroid formulas. In supplement form, this plant assists the body in producing T3 thyroid hormone[124]. Blue Flag has also exhibited anti-inflammatory potential[125]. The molecule Iridin found in Blue flag has been shown to support the liver, stimulate bile secretion and help break down fats in the body[126].
Pregnant and nursing women, as well as those suffering from hyperthyroidism should not use Blue Flag.

Guggul Myrrh (commiphora molmol)
Dose: 50mg
Guggul comes from the flowering myrrh tree in India. Guggul is actually made from the sap or gum resin of the tree. The use of guggul in Ayurvedic Medicine dates back to 600BC. In modern medicine, it is often sold in supplement form for its anti-inflammatory, anti-tumour, weight loss, thyroid stimulating and

cholesterol lowering ability[127].

Guggul contains plant sterols which have been shown to lower triglycerides and cholesterol in the body; ultimately preventing atherosclerosis (the hardening of the arteries)[128].

When it comes to hypothyroidism this gummy resin boosts thyroid function. Guggul does this by increasing the amount of iodine taken up by the thyroid gland[129]. As we discussed earlier, iodine is a key component in both thyroid hormones T3 and T4. Additionally, Guggul has also been found to increase T3 production by boosting the activity of an enzyme called thyroid peroxidase[130]. Thyroid peroxidase is the enzyme that breaks down iodide to form iodine. This iodine then attaches to tyrosine to produce T3 and T4 thyroid hormones.

Side effects from taking Guggul may include a hypersensitivity or allergic reaction which could result in skin rashes[131]. Taking too much Guggul may cause liver toxicity or even muscle wasting. This plant is not recommended for use during pregnancy.

Selenium
Dose: 55-200 micrograms
The trace element selenium can be found in many vitamin and thyroid supplements. It is even added to baby formula. In supplements, selenium often comes in the form of selenomethionine which is formed by plants. Selenium can be found in foods such as fish, Brazil nuts, peas, lentils and cereals.

Selenium yeast is another form of selenium you can buy. It is made by growing yeast in an environment where there is selenium. The non-harmful yeast binds to the selenium and then the yeast are added to supplements.

Research has shown us that selenium can act as an antioxidant. This means that it protects the body from damage caused by dangerous molecules and toxins, called free radicals. Selenium is a key antioxidant because it is a component of two major antioxidant enzymes in the body called glutathione peroxidase and thioredoxin reductase[132].

Selenium is also found in three enzymes in the body that turn thyroid hormones on and off[133]. These enzymes are called deiodinase enzymes. Hence, selenium is essential for the conversion of T4 into T3. Overall, it is a key player in normal thyroid hormone metabolism. Some studies have even found selenium supplementation to decrease thyroid peroxidase antibody count in patients[134].

Copper
Dose: 0-900 micrograms
Copper can be found in many thyroid supplements that your local health food store may carry. Often it is called copper citrate or copper malate on the label. This mineral is found in seafood, nuts, seeds, organ meats, and cocoa.

Copper deficiency is very rare in Western society. It is highly debated whether a person should take copper supplements when there are no signs of severe deficiency. Many doctors worry about their patients taking too much and suffering from copper toxicity.
Besides assisting with the treatment of osteoarthritis and wound healing, copper has been linked to thyroid function. One animal study found that low copper levels were linked to low T4 thyroid hormone levels[135]. In more recent human studies, higher blood copper levels were associated with higher T4 levels in males and a higher T3 and T4 level in females[136].

Zinc
Dose: 5mg-8 mg
Zinc, like selenium is another element that plays a role in thyroid metabolism. A recent experiment published by the American College of Nutrition found overweight, hypothyroid women who were given zinc supplements experienced a significant increase in their T3 hormone production[137].
When studying hair loss caused by hypothyroidism, scientists found zinc deficiency to also play a role[138]. This makes sense as

zinc is used in the creation of thyroid hormones. Also thyroid hormones help the body absorb zinc. So when thyroid hormone levels are low (hypothyroidism) there can be a zinc deficiency over time. These scientists also noted that hypothyroid patients prescribed thyroxine (thyroid hormone therapy) may not see their hair loss improve unless zinc supplements were also added to their treatment protocols.

Manganese
Dose: 200-500 micrograms
Manganese (not to be confused with magnesium) is another mineral used in thyroid hormone production. Daily intake of manganese may come from eating nuts, seeds, leafy green vegetables, whole grains and lentils.

Manganese forms an important antioxidant enzyme in the body called Manganese Superoxide Dimutase (MD-SOD). This mineral is found in many thyroid supplements; as a deficiency of manganese may lead to hypothyroidism[139]. However, too much manganese, even doses which are only slightly higher at the recommended amount may lead to thyroid dysfunction. If a patient were to dangerously consume greater than 11mg of manganese per day, this could cause great harm to the body.

When choosing the right thyroid formula to treat your hypothyroid and fibromyalgia symptoms, remember to follow the advice of your Naturopathic Doctor or Medical Doctor. When taking natural thyroid boosting supplements the same pharmaceutical rules apply. Be mindful of overstimulation of the thyroid as this is still a possibility when configuring your dose.
During my battle with fibromyalgia, obesity and lowered metabolism, I learned firsthand how important it is to balance stress hormone levels. In addition to thyroid therapy, these cortisol levels and the adrenal glands must be regulated. Adrenal support is a cornerstone in every good fibromyalgia protocol.

ADRENALS

It is no secret that people going through chronic stress have higher cortisol (stress hormone) levels. However, did you know that the same has been found for patients who suffer from severe chronic pain such as fibromyalgia[140]? That's right; people with chronic pain have been found to have higher cortisol levels too.

Fibromyalgia is deeply linked to mood and stress. Similarly, in patients with major depression we also see an abnormal cortisol production[141]. Fibromyalgic patients may experience anxiety, poor sleep quality, depression and chronic stress in accompaniment to their pain. When we are depressed and stressed over a long period of time our body can no longer produce enough endorphins (natural pain relieving molecules). This can result in a vicious cycle of feeling even more stressed and even more pain! Some key fibromyalgia therapy targets exist here.

First, we must lower the high stress-hormone levels. Chronic stress can make endocrine issues worst and wreak havoc on our thyroid and adrenal health[142]. Regulating this cortisol will be an important component of healing. We will focus on this approach throughout the following chapter.

Secondly, we must increase the endorphins that are naturally produced in our body in order to lower our pain perception. In a scientific study patients were injected with beta endorphin, a pain reducing opioid hormone that is created in the human brain. After receiving the endorphins their cortisol levels went down[143]. This further highlights the deep link between stress and pain.

<u>Relora</u>

<u>Source</u>: Magnolia officinalis and Phellodendron amurense
<u>Dose</u>: 300mg-900mg.

For centuries, two Chinese herbs called Magnolia officinalis and Phellodendron amurense have been used to manage stress, anxiety and poor sleep quality. In the West, these herbs have been patented into a supplement called Relora. This herbal formula can be purchased at many health food stores and pharmacies worldwide.

Have you ever been so tired and emotionally upset that you eat an entire bag of chips? How about a whole cheesecake? Well, that used to be me for a period in time before I found Relora. Recently, more and more patients are using Relora to manage weight gain caused by stress-eating.

Relora is a core component in almost all of my fibromyalgia protocols (including my own treatment). As discussed earlier, an increased or imbalanced stress hormone (cortisol) level can have very negative effects on our health. The Magnolia officinalis in Relora contains a medicinal molecule called honokiol. While the Phellodendron in Relora contains a molecule called berberine. When combined these two substances are very effective at balancing stress hormone levels. Being able to decrease our perceived daily stress and the anxiety in our body can do wonders in the recovery of fibromyalgia.

In one experiment, patients who took Relora for a month had way lower cortisol levels that those who did not take this herbal supplement[144]. These patients who took Relora also reported less stress, anger, depression and fatigue post treatment. Various animal studies have also shown that the components of Relora act similarly to anti-anxiety medications called benzodiazepines (Xanax, Valium), but without the same level of side-effects[145].

Most adults will have spiking cortisol levels around 9am, 1pm and 6pm on an average day[146]. It is suggested that one capsule of Relora (300mg) be taken at 9 am followed by 2 more capsules at 1pm to target cortisol level spiking. Your Naturopathic doctor will be able to suggest the perfect dose for you.

There is no known toxicity or serious side effects reported with using this herbal patent formula. However, taking Relora may cause you to experience drowsiness for the first few days of treatment. It is suggested that you reduce your dose or discontinue taking Relora if it upsets your stomach. Relora may interact with certain anxiety drugs. Let your health care practitioner know if you are pregnant or breastfeeding or taking prescription drugs before starting Relora.

Rhodiola
Rhodiola rosea (standardized to 3% total Rosavins and min. 1% Salidroside)
Dose: 500mg

Rhodiola (Rhodiola rosea) is a flowering plant that is found in the Arctic and mountainous areas of Europe, Asia and America. Its use in herbal medicine can be traced back as far as the ancient Greeks. Rhodiola in integrative and alternative medicine is called an "adaptogen". This term refers to the herbs' ability to assist the body in adapting to prolonged stress. Rhodiola protects us from stress through various pathways. These pathways affect the hypothalamus and pituitary gland in the brain, as well as the adrenal glands in the body[147]. Without leading you down a very complicated pathway of science and physiology, I will try to elaborate on this mechanism of action.

Scientists believe that plant adaptogens increase a stress sensing protein in the body called Hsp70. This in turn, triggers two proteins called DAF-16 and JNK-1 which modulate our resistance to stress; increasing our physical performance and longevity[148].

Beyond traditional uses in herbal stress management, Rhodiola rosea has recently been used to support low mood. This may be due to a molecule it contains called salidroside. In a recent experiment consisting of 714 subjects who suffered from stress-induced mild depression, scientists held salidroside responsible for effecting neurotransmitter pathways and creating antidepressant-like actions in subjects[149].

5-HTP (L-5-Hydroxytryptophan)
Griffonia simplicifolia seed extract
Dose: 50 mg-300mg

At the beginning of this book we established that fibromyalgia patients have significantly lower serotonin levels when compared to healthy subjects[150]. Serotonin is the neurotransmitter associated with happiness. In the body this neurotransmitter plays a role in sleep regulation, pain, depression, anxiety, appetite and mood.

A neuroscience study has found that serotonin uptake increases in normal healthy patients whenever their cortisol (stress hormone) is increased. However, patients with chronic stress, anxiety and depression did not increase their uptake of the 'happy' serotonin when cortisol was increased. This study sheds further insight into the negative effect long-term stress may have on our serotonin levels and overall mood[151].

Various international scientific journals have supported research on supplements such as 5-hydroxytryptophan (5-HTP) in the management of stress and anxiety[152]. In the body, an amino acid from our food called tryptophan is converted into 5-hydroxytryptophan (5-HTP). This 5HTP is then converted into the neurotransmitter serotonin and then into the hormone melatonin.   5-HTP supplements are extracted from seeds that come from a shrub found growing in Central Africa called Griffonia simplicifolia. Think of 5-HTP as a construction workers' toolbox. A toolbox that contains all of the components needed to build serotonin. 5-HTP is not serotonin. In fact, serotonin itself as a supplement would not be able to pass the blood-brain barrier and enter the central nervous system. 5-HTP in supplement form is well absorbed orally and once in the blood stream, 5-HTP can easily move across to the brain where it is used to produce the serotonin we are lacking[153].

Clinical trials with fibromyalgia patients have shown an improvement with 5-HTP supplementation[154]. These fibromyalgic patients reported a reduction in pain, morning stiffness, fatigue and anxiety after taking the serotonin precursor 5HTP[155]. Additionally, 5-HTP has been prescribed as a natural treatment in reducing headaches and migraines[156].

Researchers have also found 5-HTP to be effective when used in the treatment of depression[157], sleep disorders such as insomnia[158] and even weight loss[159]. This weight loss seen among obese adults after supplementation is not surprising, as 5-HTP levels have been linked to increased sugar cravings[160].

A common dose of 5-HTP prescribed to fibromyalgia patients is 50mg to 100mg three times a day. It can take up to 14 days before any effect or change is noticed. Despite this, 5-HTP-should be supplemented slowly. Starting at a low amount and increasing the dose progressively will help to minimize any side effects. Once the 5-HTP has begun to work, a reduced dosing and maintenance plan can be created with your doctor. Most of the adverse reactions to 5-HTP have been short-lived or limited. Some people may experience diarrhea, vomiting, nausea, and stomach pain. 5-HTP supplementation may cause you to feel drowsiness.

5-HTP interacts with a lot of pharmaceutical and natural drugs. Do not use 5-HTP if you are taking Carbidopa, which is prescribed for Parkinson's disease. Do not take 5-HTP with any other serotonin modulating substances. These include: Antidepressants, some pain killers (tramadol), cold medication containing dextromethorphan, migraine medication (sumatriptan), some anti-nausea medications; St. John's Wort and SAMe. Do not take 5-HTP if you are pregnant or trying to get pregnant, breastfeeding, or have a skin disease called scleroderma. Stop taking 5-HTP and see your doctor if you get skin changes, ulcers in the mouth, severe muscle and/or abdominal pain.

Melatonin
Dose: 0.3mg-5mg
Melatonin is often called the 'sleepy hormone'. It is produced in our brain and regulated by our exposure to light. In the average adult, melatonin will rise around 8:30 pm at night[161]. These

levels rise to make us sleepy. However, if we are looking at our electronic devices or in an environment with bright lights, our melatonin levels can decline. I often suggest my patients follow a sleep hygiene routine. This is where they turn off all electronics by 9pm and simply read a book, listen to music or meditate in a dimly lit room in preparation for quality sleep.

In animal studies, sleep deprivation was found to create an increase in nerve pain[162]. These studies suggest that melatonin supplements may restore a 24-hour sleep-wake cycle called circadian rhythm; while also decreasing hypersensitivity to nerve pain. Disordered sleep is common when living with fibromyalgia syndrome. Luckily, a synthetic, lab produced melatonin exists in the health market. It can be taken in supplement form and may assist with insomnia (by shortening the time it takes to fall asleep) and poor quality sleep (by reducing the amount of times we awaken during the night).

In a recent 10 day study, melatonin was given to fibromyalgia patients at bed time. Scientists found that melatonin decreased these patients' cortisol levels[163]. In this study, melatonin was also found to improve fibromyalgic pain, anxiety and overall mood.

Consequently, melatonin has been found to not only improve sleep quality but also decrease pain and pain sensitivity in fibromyalgia patients[164]. Additionally, circadian rhythms are disordered in most chronic pain syndromes; by normalizing sleep we allow for better stress management and resiliency[165].

Melatonin supplementation should be taken at night, 20 minutes before your desired bed time. Follow the dosing prescribed by your doctor. It is better to start by taking a low amount and then gradually increase your dose to an effective amount. Each patient will thrive at a different tolerated dose. Patients who are on blood thinners or blood pressure medications (for example ACE inhibitors) should avoid taking melatonin. Melatonin can affect blood sugar and is not recommended to take if you have diabetes. Melatonin may increase the risk of seizures in people who have a seizure disorder. Melatonin is not recommended for patients who are on immuno-suppressant drugs. Melatonin may cause drowsiness. It may also worsen depression symptoms in some people.

GABA (gamma-Aminobutyric acid)
Dose: 250mg-750mg
AND
Glycine
Dose: 1000mg-15g

Currently, there isn't much research out there supporting the use of GABA and glycine for pain. Despite the lack of clinical trials, I have had profound results taking them both. I have also had positive feedback from many other fibromyalgic patients who combine these supplements to help with various stress symptoms.

GABA (gamma-Aminobutyric acid) is a chemical messenger that is made in the brain. GABA acts as a neurotransmitter by signalling our neurons to calm down. This is why GABA is often referred to as an 'inhibitory neurotransmitter' which can relax our stressed out, over-excited brains[166]. Doctors found that stressed-out patients who took GABA in an oral supplement form had changes to their brain waves within an hour[167]. This resulted in increased relaxation and lowered anxiety.

As discussed before, stress and adrenal fatigue can cause many changes in our bodies. One proposed negative change among fibromyalgia sufferers may involve our neurotransmitters. These are the molecules our nerves use to communicate with each other, such as dopamine, serotonin and GABA. In fact, researchers have found an area in the brain where GABA levels are much lower among fibromyalgia patients (when compared to healthy people)[168]. For anyone interested in specifics, this area of the brain is called the right anterior insula.

GABA plays a key role in regulating how the human brain experiences anxiety[169]. A poor regulation of GABA level is linked to anxiety disorders. For example, one brain imaging study discovered that people who suffer from post-traumatic stress disorder also have abnormally reduced levels of GABA in the right anterior insula[170]. Similar reductions in GABA levels have been viewed in patients suffering from panic disorder too[171]. Finally, sleep studies have also shown that non-medicated patients who suffer from insomnia exhibit 30% reduced brain GABA levels[172].

At this point you may be wondering why every fibromyalgia sufferer doesn't take GABA. This is where things get complicated. Fibromyalgia is such a complex disease that even though there are dysfunctional changes with our transmitter systems, these changes do not occur uniformly among all patients. Every patient is different. Some fibromyalgia patients might find that GABA and glycine really help to block their over-excited brain signals. Others may find this approach overly sedative or ineffective. This is why we must explore every treatment option in order to enable you and your doctor to create a plan that is specific to your needs.

Despite the lack of extensive research on GABA supplements there have been reported improvements to pain, fatigue and poor sleep in the clinical trials of pharmaceuticals drugs which turn on and attach to GABA receptors; as well as with studies of benzodiazepines which enhance the effect of GABA in the body[173]. Unfortunately, many people taking GABA orally may not notice huge effects right away. This is because supplemented GABA does not cross the blood brain barrier (BBB) very easily. To help GABA get into the brain and decrease excitability, a substance called glycine is also often taken with it.

Glycine is an amino acid that helps with protein creation in the body. Glycine also acts as a neurotransmitter in the brain and spine. Like GABA, glycine has the ability to calm down nerves in an over-excited brain which assists in improving sleep and stress[174].

It is important to note that neuroscientists have also discovered a vitamin B6 deficiency can cause the body to produce lower GABA levels[175]. This is due to the fact that vitamin B6 helps an enzyme in our neurons make GABA. We will discuss the importance of B vitamins for fibromyalgia syndrome later in this book.

GABA and glycine should not be taken for long periods of time. It is important to speak to your Naturopathic Doctor if taking them for longer than 6 weeks. It is best to avoid taking both these supplements if you are pregnant or breastfeeding. GABA can reduce blood pressure. Caution must be taken if you are also taking blood pressure lowering pharmaceuticals or supplements.

Now that we have discussed various methods of approaching stress, mood and sleep dysfunction, let's get into our Fibromyalgia Pain Protocol!

PAIN PROTOCOL

Magnesium Malate

Sourced from Magnesium and Malic Acid

Dose: 100mg-300mg Elemental Magnesium + 540mg-1500mg Malic Acid

Magnesium is an element involved in hundreds of our bodily processes. These include energy creation and the relaxation of muscles. Researchers have also found that magnesium blocks a pain receptor called NMDA in the body[176].When the NMDA pain receptor is activated we can experience more pain via sensory pathways in the brain and spine. The activity of NMDA pain receptors has been found to be increased in fibromyalgia syndrome[177]. Hence, magnesium is a key therapeutic intervention when it comes to pain management.

Fibromyalgia patients have much lower red blood cell magnesium levels when compared to osteoarthritis patients[178]. Various studies have linked this magnesium deficiency to muscle pain among fibromyalgic patients[179]. Furthermore, patients with chronic fatigue syndrome who also have low red blood cell magnesium levels report increased energy levels, lower pain and better mood when treated with magnesium[180].

The big question here is: Why do these magnesium abnormalities exist in some fibromyalgia sufferers? One potential answer is diet. Magnesium is found in many food sources, such as green veggies, seeds, nuts, whole grains and even chocolate. Magnesium also plays a role in allowing us to absorb other nutrients from our food. However, a Western diet rich in tea, coffee, alcohol and even refined flour (white bread and pasta) can all work against us, by depleting our body's magnesium levels.

Another possible cause for low magnesium levels may be low ATP. ATP is a molecule in the body that stores and transports energy. Scientists in the past have suggested that fibromyalgia patients may have a heightened demand by their body to make more ATP. Magnesium malate plays an important role in this ATP energy production[181]. When left untreated, this energy demand can even result in the undesired breakdown of muscles. This muscle protein is then used to create energy.

Magnesium in the form of magnesium malate is created by combining the element magnesium with malic acid. Malic acid is an organic compound naturally made in our bodies. Magnesium malate in supplement form can be taken with food, and has been shown to be easily absorbed. The theory is that magnesium malate is excellent for supporting energy levels. This may be due to the fact that the malic acid it contains plays a major role in the production of ATP.

Fibromyalgia patients, who were given higher doses of magnesium malate (made of 300mg magnesium and 1200mg malic acid) responded positively, with major reductions in pain and tenderness after only 2 months of supplementation[182].

When it comes to your individual fibromyalgia protocol, you may need more or less magnesium malate. Consult your physician and discontinue if pregnant or lactating. It is important to speak to your doctor if you are taking any medication that may interact with magnesium.

Fish Oil- Omega-3 Essential Fatty Acids
Sourced from anchovies, sardines and/or mackerel
Dose: 1200mg to 3000mg of Omega-3 EFA (750mg-2000mg EPA and 500-1000mg DHA)
Omega-3 fish oil supplements contain two therapeutic fatty acids called Eicosapentaenoic acid (EPA) and Docosahexaenoic acid (DHA). These are of particular interest to us when creating an anti-inflammatory fibromyalgia protocol.

Researchers have found that these essential fatty acids may play a role in limiting the genes that control inflammation in the body[183]. They also inhibit pro-inflammatory molecules called eicosanoids and have been found to decrease nerve pain in patients[184]. A scientific experiment found 60% of patients with neck and back pain who took 1200mg of omega-3 essential fatty acids (in the form of fish oil supplements) reported an overall pain improvement within one month[185]. As a result, 59% of the patients in this study were also able to stop taking their prescription anti-inflammatory drugs.

Beyond influencing pain and inflammation, omega-3 fish oils have been found to benefit patients with cardiovascular disease, support the human brain and eyes and even modulate our immune system[186].

I like to think of the "P" in EPA as "Pain"; and the "H" in DHA as "Head". This helps me remember that DHA plays an incredibly important role in the development of our brains from the moment we are developing in the womb[187]. When DHA is deficient, we see reduced growth with poor eye and brain development in kids.

DHA may even help with brain injury. Traumatic brain injury is something I experienced first-hand via my car accident. This was followed by a concussion and post-concussion syndrome. Beyond headaches, light sensitivity and dizziness, I also had memory deficits and migraines. In retrospect, I wish I had known a whole body of research supporting the dietary supplementation of essential fatty acids existed. One study actually found that DHA reduced the intensity at which our body experienced a traumatic brain injury[188]. This pain and brain connection is further emphasized in patients who showed greater levels of serotonin blood markers when taking omega-3 supplements[189]. Recently, scientists were amazed to learn that altering omega-3 intake may even improve psychological distress among individuals who suffer from chronic headaches[190]. Similar positive mood outcomes were found when omega-3 essential fatty acids improved major depression[191] as well as lowered anxiety levels in research patients[192].

When it comes to fibromyalgia syndrome, many patients also suffer from chronic fatigue and irritable bowel syndrome (IBS)[193]. There is so much new research exploring how our gut is connected to our brain; with some doctors even suggesting that a healthy gut is the key to our ultimate wellbeing. When the good and bad bacteria in our gut become imbalanced this is called dysbiosis. Dysbiosis of various gut bacteria has been found in IBS patients. It has been established that omega-3 fatty acids may positively influence our gut bacteria composition[194]. This is another compelling reason for incorporating this supplement into a fibromyalgia pain protocol.

You may be wondering if you can skip taking fish oil supplements altogether and just eat fish. Well, you definitely can. However, there are a couple things to keep in mind. Firstly, the American Heart Association recommends eating ¾ cup of flaked fatty fish or 3.5 oz of fish at a minimum intake of twice a week. Depending on the level of cardiovascular disease the EPA and DHA intake recommended varies from 1-4 grams per day[195]. It can be very difficult to reach these therapeutic doses with a dietary intake of fatty fish alone. Secondly, the fish that are high in omega-3 fatty acids include salmon, mackerel, trout, herring, albacore tuna and sardines. Unfortunately, many of these fish can accumulate toxic levels of heavy metals. Eating them in excessive abundance (more than 2-3 times a week) may not be safe. Hence, at 40-80 calories per serving, a high grade, filtered fish oil supplement in addition to a fish dinner once or twice a week, may be a more appropriate choice. For more consumer information on fatty fish and heavy metal toxicity you can check out the Environmental Working Group at www.ewg.org.

Glucosamine (d-glucosamine HCL) + Chondroitin (chondroitin sulfate sodium) and MSM (methylsulfonylmethanean)
Sources: Shrimp, crab or other shellfish exoskeleton (glucosamine); Bovine/porcine or avian cartilage (chondroitin); Laboratory produced (MSM).

<u>Dose</u>: 1500mg Glucosamine + 1200mg Chondroitin + 900mg MSM per day for a minimum of three months.

I debated writing about these three popular supplements which are often taken together. There is much argument and conflicting research regarding their use among the medical community. Having suffered from intense knee pain as a result of a car accident and a worsening of this pain throughout fibromyalgia flare ups, glucosamine, chondroitin and MSM at the therapeutic doses outlined above helped me immensely.

One six month study published in the journal of *Arthritis and Rheumatology* found no improvement on joint pain or function among patients taking glucosamine and chondroitin sulfate[196]. Whereas, another research paper published in the same year, noted an overall benefit among patients with knee pain and stiffness when they were supplemented with glucosamine-chondroitin sulfate and MSM[197].

As you can see there is no concrete scientific evidence ensuring the efficacy of this supplement for knee pain. Regardless, there have still been many compelling studies supporting their use.

So, despite the existence of some clinical trials rendering the above supplements ineffective with pain reduction, I will be focusing on those studies that instead support them.

Glucosamine is believed by some to assist in cartilage repair. This may be due its sulfur content. Sulfur plays a role in cartilage building. Cartilage is the rubber like tissue that cushions our joints. After a month of giving patients with osteoarthritis knee pain 1500mg of glucosamine sulfate; researchers noted that these patients had a similar improvement of their joint pain and function compared to those patients who instead took ibuprofen (non-steroidal anti-inflammatory drugs)[198]. A more compelling three year study, exhibited joint stiffness, knee pain and physical mobility improvements among patients taking glucosamine sulfate as a means to delay the progression of osteoarthritis in the knee[199].

Similarly, research has established that chondroitin sulfate improved knee pain faster in patients after six to nine months of consistent therapy[200]. When compared to the anti-inflammatory drug Celecoxib, both chondroitin and glucosamine reduced joint space narrowing and produced less gastrointestinal (stomach) upset among patients[201].

MSM (methylsulfonylmethane) is an organic sulphur containing compound that naturally exists. It is often marketed and used as an anti-inflammatory agent. MSM can also be found as a component in various natural topical pain creams. Research has indicated that MSM may improve joint and muscle pain, as well decrease inflammation[202]. One investigative study found that an orally supplemented combination of glucosamine and MSM reduced not only joint pain, but also swelling; this enhanced the functioning of patients[203].

It is important to seek physician guidance if pregnant or breast-feeding before beginning this combination therapy for joint pain. Also, the above supplements may cause bloating, indigestion and/or constipation in some individuals. It is recommended to check in with your health care provider every 3 months to monitor physical progress and dosing once you begin therapy with glucosamine, chondroitin and MSM

Cannabis (Medical Marijuana)
Source: Flowering plant
Dose: Dosing varies from patient to patient.
Medical Cannabis (medical marijuana) has recently been gaining clout among the medical community. This may be a reflection of the global progress in cannabis research, as well as the legalization of medical and recreational marijuana in some countries and states. Currently, there is an abundant array of scientific evidence supporting the use of medical marijuana for chronic nerve pain[204].
The cannabis plant has over 483 compounds. These include

the psychoactive compound tetrahydrocannabinol (THC) that can make a person feel "high" and the non-psychotropic cannabidiol (CBD). Bothe these compounds work on the endo-cannabinoid receptors located in our nervous and immune systems[205]. Some common conditions where physicians may prescribe medical cannabis include arthritis, chronic pain, headache and migraine[206].

An article published in the *European Journal of Pain* noted a decreased sensitivity to nerve pain, as well as an overall improvement on well-being and mood, among patients who were treated with cannabinoids[207]. There is some debate as to whether this positive improvement in mood is actually the cause of the decreased nerve pain perception in patients.

In animal studies, CBD (the non-psychoactive component of cannabis) has been shown to suppress inflammatory nerve pain by playing a role in the "nociceptive" or pain sensory centers of the spine[208]. When it comes to decreasing that burning and spasm-like muscle pain in humans, medical cannabis has shown great promise[209]. Even among patients whose pain was not relieved by strong opioid drugs, scientists found that combination THC and CBD extracts were able to provide pain relief[210]. Rheumatology research has consistently found cannabis to reduce non-cancer pain in patients[211]. Unfortunately, the above findings are not enough to indicate the use of medical marijuana in ALL situations of chronic, non-cancer pain, such as fibromyalgia. I must emphasize again that every fibromyalgic patient is different. It is important to speak to your doctor and decipher what dose and specific percentage of THC (psychoactive) and CBD (non-psychoactive) cannabis is appropriate for you. Some individuals may experience anxiety with THC, whereas others may notice the opposite effect. CBD may cause drowsiness in some patients. Medical marijuana, when dosed and prescribed appropriately, has been shown to be well tolerated short term. The adverse and long-term effects of this herb are not well established. The most common side-effect is dizziness; with long-term concerns ranging from poor memory to mental health issues with marijuana use among teenagers[212].

STRESS MANAGEMENT

It is imperative at this point to reiterate the importance of stress management as a key to fibromyalgia pain management. As discussed earlier, an imbalance of cortisol and an abnormally higher stress response are important contributors to fibromyalgic chronic pain[213]. Consequently, women with fibromyalgia have reported higher pain levels at the same time of day where researchers have also found higher stress hormone levels in their saliva[214]. The link between stress and pain is undeniable. This is especially true for fibromyalgia patients like me, who also suffer from post-traumatic stress disorder (PTSD). Symptoms of trauma are commonly found among fibromyalgia patients. Individuals with fibromyalgia have actually been found to experience greater negative symptoms from PTSD, when compared to those PTSD patients who do not have fibromyalgia[215]. Later in this book, we will explore other pain and stress management avenues as part of our individualized fibromyalgia protocol. These include physical therapy, meditation, acupuncture, music therapy and exercise for example.

Before we delve deeper into pain reduction, we must work towards implementing strategies to increase those low fibromyalgic energy levels.

ENERGY BOOST

Vitamin D3 (Cholecalciferol)

Sourced most commonly from the sun (exposure to skin); or lanolin (oil extracted from sheep's wool); or plant sourced from lichen (fungi, algae and cycanobacteria compounds).

Dose: 1000 IUmg-4000IU +++ (Depending on deficiency levels)

Vitamin D is a fat-soluble vitamin. Our body produces vitamin D from our skin and ultraviolet radiation (UV rays) from the sun. It is also available in a supplement form called vitamin D3 or Cholecalciferol. As discussed earlier, people living in tropical, sunny climates produce a lot more vitamin D throughout the year than their northern counterparts. You may have heard that Vitamin D is important to bone health. You may have also wondered why milk products often have vitamin D added to them. Well, this is because Vitamin D helps our body to absorb minerals such as calcium, magnesium and phosphate. Vitamin D has also been found to have anti-inflammatory properties and play a role in muscle health, making it particularly interesting within the field of fibromyalgia research[216]. It has been well established that patients who report feeling tired to their doctors may also have low vitamin D levels. After supplementing these patients with vitamin D3 and restoring their levels back to normal, there is an improvement of even severe fatigue symptoms[217].

Currently, more and more scientists are linking fibromyalgia symptom severity to a vitamin D deficiency and supporting the idea that this vitamin may improve the quality of life of fibromyalgic patients[218]. Various studies have shown low vitamin D levels among fibromyalgia patients[219]. The role of vitamin D in pain perception has been a widely explored topic. It is hypothesized that people with chronic pain and fibromyalgia may not be as mobile and receive adequate sunlight exposure.

20 weeks of oral vitamin D supplementation had a very positive effect among women with fibromyalgia syndrome, who reported decreased pain perception[220]. Similarly, a more recent study examined fibromyalgia patients between the ages of 28-67 years. These patients were also given vitamin D orally, over a course of 3 months. The published results of this study included a reduction in their overall fibromyalgia tender points post vitamin D supplementation[221]. Subsequently, it has been proposed that low levels of vitamin D may actually be a risk factor and worsen symptoms of fibromyalgia[222]. However, the exact mechanism by which vitamin D affects the nervous system pathways in fibromyalgic patients is still unknown.

Luckily, vitamin D is a relatively cheap supplement. It is easy to access with minimum side effects when taken appropriately. So how much vitamin D should we take? This is where I must refer you back to your doctor for blood work, as it really depends on a number of factors. The tolerable upper intake level for a male or female over 19 years of age is 4000IU of supplemented vitamin D per day[223]. This means the maximum amount you could take per day with no expected side effects is 4000IU of vitamin D3.

However, some of us are more or less deficient and will require more or less of this vitamin. For example, some patients are taking levels as low as 1000IU per day, whereas others are prescribed upwards of 10,000 IU per day. Also, within various disease states our liver and kidneys may not be able to handle such a high level of this fat soluble vitamin. Vitamin D overloading and toxicity can cause heart rhythm complications. Taking too much vitamin D can also raise calcium levels in the blood, leading to the hardening of blood vessels.

At this point in our discussion, you may be wondering: Why the hell does mega-dose vitamin D supplementation cause toxicity, but being in the sun with exposed skin for hours does not? This perfectly highlights the magnificence with which the human body functions naturally. Excessive sun exposure will heat up the skin. This heat on the skin breaks down the extra vitamin D as it is formed, limiting the potential for toxic levels to build up when tanning[224].

SAMe (S-adenosyl-l-methionine)
Source: Naturally made in the body. Supplement is synthesized in a laboratory.
Dose: 200mg -800mg per day.

When it comes to energy, a key player we must focus on is the mitochondria. Mitochondria are small little structures that float around every cell in our body. They provide our body with energy, in the form of a molecule called ATP. If you think of our bodies as a pinball machine, ATP would be the "energy currency" or the quarters needed for the game console to light up and work. Hence, ATP produced by the mitochondria is necessary for bodily function and metabolism on a cellular level.

S-adenosyl-l-methionine or SAMe is a supplement that is found to increase the amount of mitochondria in the cells of animals[225]. SAMe is naturally found in the human body. A lab created form of SAMe is also sold as a prescription drug or natural supplement, around the world. Besides playing a potential role in energy production, SAMe has also shown anti-depressant effects; plays a role in hormone regulation; decreases pain from osteoarthritis; and helps in the treatment of liver disease[226][227]. Upon examining the skin cells of fibromyalgia sufferers, researchers found signs of cellular stress, inflammation and surprisingly, dysfunctional mitochondria[228]. Another study which examined the muscle fibres from fibromyalgic patients also discovered abnormal mitochondria present. This included abnormal mitochondrial shape, positioning, quantity and an atypical distribution of mitochondria in the fibromyalgia patients' cells[229]. Findings of such mitochondrial defects in fibromyalgia patients, has led some scientists to postulate that this may be another missing puzzle piece in the fibromyalgia disease process[230].

When scientists gave 800mg of SAMe to fibromyalgia patients for six weeks, they found improvements in patients' fatigue, mood, morning stiffness and pain[231]. Are these reductions in fibromyalgia fatigue linked to the mitochondria changes caused by SAMe? Unfortunately, there is not enough research to answer this question conclusively. However, we do know that when we increase mitochondrial density in the cells (when we have a larger number of bigger sized mitochondria present) they can better make ATP energy for our muscles to use [232].

It has been recommended that SAMe be taken on an empty stomach; but not at night, as it may cause wakefulness/insomnia, restlessness and even anxiety in some patients. As always speak with your health care practitioner prior to use. Caution should be taken if you are pregnant, breastfeeding, or on any antidepressant medications.

At this point, I would like to touch base with you, the reader of this book. I want to applaud you for taking ownership over your health and reading through the overwhelming amount of material I have presented here, thus far. I know it is a lot of information to process and it can be intimidating. Fibromyalgia is a complicated disease. I really hope that there is new information presented here that is keeping you interested and hopeful. Also, if you are referring to the research references and taking notes throughout this journey with me, this information may be better remembered.

I want to reiterate that the purpose of this book is to equip every fibromyalgia sufferer in the world with an arsenal of effective, clinically researched, treatment options from which an individualized plan can be concocted by you and your doctor. I would be remiss to omit any information. You rock! Keep reading! We are getting closer and closer to the day you can say

F*ck Fibromyalgia!

NADH (Nicotinamide Adenine Dinucleotide)
Source: Naturally produced from Vitamin B-3 (Niacin) in the body. Supplement is synthesized in a laboratory.
Dose: 5mg-10mg per day.

You may be reading the above supplement and thinking: What the hell is NADH?! Before I was diagnosed with fibromyalgia, I had no idea this coenzyme was so readily available in supplement form at my local health food store. A coenzyme is a substance which helps certain enzymes in our body work properly. The coenzyme NADH is made from vitamin B-3 and can be found in all of our cells. Our body uses NADH for many important biological processes; including the production of ATP energy.

Low energy and extreme tiredness is a common symptom of chronic fatigue syndrome and fibromyalgia. As discussed above, abnormal levels of ATP in the cells may be a reason for this poor energy production; which is why researchers have examined NADH as an energy booster[233]. In an experiment where patients with chronic fatigue were given 10mg of NADH a day, for four weeks, 31% responded positively with a betterment of symptoms; when compared to the patients who received a placebo (fake treatment) instead[234]. A more extensive study found chronic fatigue syndrome patients who were given NADH, experienced a significant lessening of their symptoms within 8 months. This included a lower intensity of fatigue and decreased anxiety. Furthermore, these patients continued to improve over the following year post-treatment[235].

Often NADH is prescribed with another coenzyme called CoQ10. When taken together, these supplements have been found to reduce the perception of fatigue among patients with chronic fatigue syndrome[236]. Researchers exploring these potential energy boosters learned that chronic fatigue patients taking 20mg/day of NADH and 200mg/day of CoQ10 had increased ATP levels within an 8 week trial period[237].

Coenzyme Q10 (CoQ10, ubiquinone, ubiquinol)
Source: Naturally produced in the body. Found in some foods. Supplement is synthesized in a laboratory.
Dose: 100mg-200mg per day.

Another coenzyme or "enzyme helper" that exists in our body is called coenzyme Q10 (CoQ10). Coenzyme Q10 exists in different biochemical forms in the body, known as ubiquinol or ubiquinone. Our bodies naturally produce Coenzyme Q10, but its production may decrease in certain diseases or even as we age.

CoQ10 can be found in various foods including organ meats, fatty fish, broccoli, spinach, cauliflower, lentils and sesame seeds, to name a few. It acts as an antioxidant and assists in protecting and supporting the mitochondria[238]. Basically, CoQ10 helps the mitochondria make ATP. Remember, the mitochondria in our cells function to produce ATP energy currency from the carbohydrates and fats we eat. So when CoQ10 is missing, the amount of ATP produced by the mitochondria reduces[239].

Like mitochondria dysfunction, CoQ10 deficiency has been linked to fibromyalgia. In an attempt to better understand this link between mitochondrial dysfunction, fibromyalgia and low CoQ10, scientists further examined the cells of fibromyalgic patients. One published paper describes how a fibromyalgic woman (who unsurprisingly also had low CoQ10 levels) was able to restore her cells' irregular mitochondrial functioning by taking this supplement[240].

When scientists gave fibromyalgia patients 300mg/day of CoQ10 supplements for 40 days, they found increased mitochondria levels in their cells[241]. After this CoQ10 treatment, researchers also found that these patients had a reduction of the following symptoms: fatigue, morning tiredness, tender points and pain[242]. Similarly, a Spanish study on fibromyalgia patients, found a reduction in trigger point pain levels and an increase in overall energy after oral coenzyme Q10 therapy[243]. Even in studies of children suffering from fibromyalgia with low CoQ10 levels, ubiquinol supplements were shown to reduce symptoms of fatigue as well as normalize cholesterol levels[244].

As mentioned above, coenzyme Q10 can be found in different forms in the body. There are two forms of CoQ10 found in supplements. When you read the labels at your local pharmacy you may see CoQ10 in the form of ubiquinone or ubiquinol. Research has shown that the ubiquinol form of CoQ10 is better absorbed in the gut; this results in a greater activation of mitochondria functioning, leading to ATP energy production[245]. This is why ubiquinol supplements may cost more money than the ubiquinone ones. To offset this issue, some companies add black pepper to their ubiquinone formulations to simulate the gut and create better absorption of this CoQ10 form.

D-Ribose (beta-d-ribofuranose, D-ribosa, ribose)
Source: Naturally produced in the body.
Dose: 5g-15g per day.
D-ribose is substance naturally found in our bodies. Its structure looks similar to sugar. It is made by our cells and used by the mitochondria to produce ATP. The heart produces D-ribose but with decreased blood flow and oxygen, this production can slow down. This may result in low ATP production. D-ribose enhances ATP production[246]. When the heart muscle cells don't have ATP energy they can't do their job and function properly. Hence, D-ribose is often prescribed to patients suffering from cardiovascular diseases. Often, athletes are also prescribed ribose by their Naturopathic Doctor, to boost muscle energy and improve exercise tolerance.
An interesting case study examined the effects of adding D-ribose to the treatment regimen of a fibromyalgic woman. Researchers found that she had a resulting improvement of her fibromyalgia symptoms and as a result, they noted ribose may help to improve energy metabolism for similar patients[247].

This finding was further emphasized two years later, in a larger study consisting of fibromyalgia and chronic fatigue syndrome patients. In this experiment, 41 of these patients were given D-ribose at a dose of 5g three times a day; after 3 weeks of this treatment patients reported increased energy, better sleep, less mental fogginess and lower pain levels[248].

An article published in the *Journal of Integrative Medicine* suggests taking 5g of D-ribose, 3 times per day, for 6 weeks and then reducing this dose to 5g, twice per day for an additional 6 weeks[249]. This progressive decrease in dosing is because long term safety has yet to be established. However, ribose has generally been considered safe with short term use. Some side-effects may include: headache, diarrhea, a feeling of being wired or overly-energized, and low blood sugar. As always, speak to your doctor, as D-ribose can interact with alcohol, aspirin and various medications which can all lead to a drastic drop in blood sugar levels.

Acetyl-L-carnitine
Source: Naturally produced in the body.
Dose: 500mg-2000mg per day.
When it comes to energy production in the body, L-carnitine is another important game player. L-carnitine is an amino acid (protein builder) that is naturally produced in our bodies. L-carnitine can also be acquired from eating red meat. This compound plays a part in moving fatty acids to the mitochondria, where these fats are burned to create usable ATP energy[250].

This supplement is available in two forms: L-carnitine and acetyl-L-carnitine. Even though they work similarly, oral acetyl-L-carnitine has been found to absorb better in the gut[251]. In diabetic patients, with nerve damage, researchers found acetyl-l-carnitine helped the damaged nerve fibers heal and grow, within the course of 1 year[252]. Similarly, patients with diabetic nerve damage also had a decrease in pain with acetyl-l-carnitine supplementation[253].

In elderly patients, acetyl-L-carnitine was not only found to improve brain functioning,[254] but also reduced fatigue[255]. Subsequently, fibromyalgia research has showed some promising results with this "mitochondria booster". In one study, 152 fibromyalgic patients were given 500mg to 1000mg of acetyl-L-carnitine for 10 weeks; they reported lower pain and stiffness levels; and experienced reduced fatigue with decreased feelings of tiredness when waking up in the morning[256]. When compared to the antidepressant Cymbalta (duloxetine), acetyl-l-carnitine was found to have similar positive effects on physical pain, energy and depression among fibromyalgia patients[257].

There are fewer side effects from taking acetyl-l-carnitine orally vs. taking it through an IV drip. Some people who take this supplement may notice a fishy odour in their pee, sweat or breath. It is important to take the amount recommended by your doctor and start supplementing with a low dose (500mg) first. Limiting treatment to one year may be advantageous, as long-term safety has not yet been established. Some people may experience nausea, stomach pain, vomiting and restlessness with acetyl-l-carnitine use[258].

We all know that fatigue is such a large theme during our fibromyalgia patient experience. Patients report feelings of physical tiredness, emotional fatigue and low motivation, as well as, mental fog or cognitive exhaustion[259]. Increasing ATP cellular energy and fixing dysfunctional mitochondria is one vital approach. However, fixing vitamin deficiencies in the body may be another preferred treatment method.

VITAL VITAMINS

<u>Vitamin C (ascorbic acid, L-ascorbic acid)</u>

<u>Source</u>: Fruits and vegetables. Supplements are also sourced from food extracts or lab created.

<u>Dose</u>: 500mg-2000mg+ per day.

"Are you eating enough servings of raw fruits and vegetables?" my mother always asked. It was not until my mid 20's that I really started to appreciate organic fruit and veggie smoothies. They truly make me feel invincible!

Vitamin C is a water soluble vitamin that comes from fruits and vegetables. Raw meat can also contain vitamin C, but this is all destroyed during cooking[260]. In fact, cooking vegetables via steaming, grilling and boiling can cause a 22-60% loss of vitamin C[261]. Unlike the fat soluble vitamins (A, D, E and K), our body is not very good at storing water soluble vitamins and we must obtain them from our daily diet.

Vitamin C is essential to a proper functioning body. It plays a role in the production of collagen, cholesterol, catecholamines (such as dopamine and epinephrine) and even L-carnitine[262]. We just discussed the importance of carnitine and energy. Well, vitamin C helps activate the enzymes that make carnitine in our cells[263]. Yet, researchers are still trying to figure out the specifics of how a vitamin C deficiency may lead to altered carnitine production. It is not surprising to learn that symptoms of low mood and fatigue are often reported by patients in the early stages of vitamin C deficiency[264].

Vitamin C deficiencies have also been linked to neck and back pain, as well as arthritis[265]. Some scientists suggest that vitamin C may be a good add-on therapy for pain relief[266]. This is because vitamin C has been found to decrease inflammation in the body[267].

Vitamin C at a dose of 500mg per day for 2 weeks was also found to decrease anxiety in students[268]. Demonstrating again, the positive effect regularly eating fruits and vegetables can have on our mind and body.

Unfortunately, smokers have lower vitamin C levels when compared to non-smokers, who consume the same amount of fruits and vegetables as them. As smoking depletes vitamin C, some researchers recommend smokers should intake a slightly higher amount of daily vitamin C[269]. When assessing how much vitamin C is necessary in our daily diet, we must keep in mind that vitamin C status will vary among healthy patients versus those in a disease state. Some of us will have more or less of a need for these ascorbic acid supplements.

Vitamin C is pretty well tolerated, even at doses of 1000mg to 2000mg. However, ingesting too much supplemental vitamin C may cause stomach pain, diarrhea, trouble sleeping, flushed skin and headache[270]. To counteract this, some doctors will administer a high dose of vitamin C intravenously, instead of orally. Also, because vitamin C is water soluble, our body can only absorb and use so much of the oral supplement before we pee it out. The recommended daily amount for vitamin C maintenance in <u>healthy</u> individuals is around 75mg for adult women and 90mg for men[271].

B-Vitamins (B1, B2, B3, B5, B6, B7, B9 and B12)
<u>Source</u>: Various Food Sources.
<u>Dose</u>: Varies
The 8-soluble, B-vitamins are essential to health. It would take another 100 pages to write about all of the roles these B-vitamins play in our body. From energy production, metabolism and thyroid function, to DNA repair, to the communication between neurons, these vitamins are in some way involved[272]. Deficiencies in B vitamins have been linked to muscle pain[273].

In this section of the book, we will briefly discuss each B-vitamin and the role they play in our fibromyalgia protocol. Globally, these vitamins can be purchased individually or together in capsule form as a B-complex supplement. Your Naturopathic Doctor can also administer a B-complex through an injection into the muscle or intravenously via an IV drip formula known as the Myers Cocktail.

Vitamin B1 (Thiamine)

Source: Seeds and nuts, eggs yolks, beef liver, pork, broccoli, peas, oranges, oats and fortified (added to) rice, cereal, pasta and breads.

Dose: 50mg-100mg

A vitamin B1 (Thiamine) deficiency is known as beriberi. This can occur among people with a poor diet and genetic issues. Beriberi can also be present in certain disease states, like cancer and diabetes for example.

Vitamin B1 helps our body convert carbohydrates from our diet into energy for our brain and muscles. This vitamin also plays a role in muscle function and communication between our nerves[274]. When it comes to medicine, there is a lot of promising research underway on thiamine use.

Scientists have found that B1 helps prolong pain-reduction when added to local anaesthetics in surgery[275]. Similar to fibromyalgia symptoms, individuals suffering from a thiamine deficiency may also experience muscle weakness and pain, irritable bowels, headaches, poor mood and sleep issues[276]. As a result, some doctors believe that there could be a vitamin B1 deficiency and fibromyalgia link. In fibromyalgia syndrome, it has been suggested that aside from a low intake of thiamine rich foods, there could be an enzyme dysfunction that is messing up thiamine transportation into the mitochondria[277].

In one study, researchers found that a high dose vitamin B1 supplement improved the symptoms of widespread pain, fatigue, dry skin and anxiety among fibromyalgia patients[278]. It is interesting to note that none of these fibromyalgia patients had any signs of thiamine deficiencies in their blood work before treatment.

High dose thiamine was also given to patients who had no thiamine deficiency on blood testing but suffered from inflammatory bowel diseases such as Crohn's and ulcerative colitis[279]. These patients noted decreased levels of chronic fatigue and tiredness.

Vitamin B2 (Riboflavin)

Source: Green vegetables; Eggs, milk, meat, mushrooms, and often added to grains.

Dose: 50mg-100mg

Vitamin B2 (Riboflavin), like the other B vitamins, is important for ATP energy production in our cells. Riboflavin helps our body to process iron and it also activates both vitamins B6 and B9 into usable forms[280].

Migraines are often a major complaint among fibromyalgia patients. Many scientists believe that migraines could be linked to dysfunctional mitochondria and ATP energy production issues in the brain[281]. Vitamin B2 has been deemed safe and effective as a preventative migraine supplement; it is believed to assist somehow in bettering energy in the brain[282].

Vitamin B3 (Niacin, nicotinic acid, niacinamide, nicotinamide riboside)

Source: Bran, yeast, poultry, red meat, eggs, yeast, fish, legumes, seeds, whole-grains.

Dose: 50mg-100mg

There are two forms of vitamin B3 (niacin). One is called niacinamide (also known as nicotinamide) and the other is called nicotinic acid[283]. Nicotinic acid when taken in supplement form can cause flushing of the skin, due to its ability to temporary widen blood vessels. This may have some positive benefits to heart health. Niacinamide (nicotinamide) is the form of B3 that does not cause flushing, yet still has other proposed health benefits. Vitamin B3 is important for energy production, as well as nerve health and development[284].

In the Energy Boost section of this book we spoke about NADH. Well, if you recall, NADH is a molecule in our body used to produce energy. The N in NADH stands for nicotinamide aka

Vitamin B3! NADH is made in our body from vitamin B3[285]. As you can see, vitamin B3 plays an important role in ATP energy production within the mitochondria of our cells[286]. In animal experiments, vitamin B3 has been found to have pain reduction and anti-inflammatory effects[287]. In one study where scientists gave patients vitamin B3 supplements for 3 weeks, the patients found a resulting decrease in insomnia and an increase in quality sleep experiences[288].

Vitamin B5 (Pantothenic acid)
Source: meat, liver, kidney, fish, chicken, eggs, milk, vegetables and legumes.
Dose: 50-100mg
Pantothenic acid (vitamin B5) assists in the processing of carbohydrates, proteins and fats from our diet. B5 also plays a role in creating the molecule that helps to create cortisol and acetylcholine in the body[289]. Cortisol and acetylcholine are important to fibromyalgia. Cortisol is our stress hormone and acetylcholine is what our nerves release in order to activate our muscles. Additionally, low pantothenic acid (B5) in the body has been linked to low immunity and inflammation[290].
In animal studies, B5 supplementation was found to increase adrenal functioning[291]. In one human study, researchers gave subjects high doses of vitamin B5 for six weeks. After this B5 therapy, the subjects exhibited a decreased drop in immune cells when they were exposed to extreme physical stress[292]. Although the specifics are unknown, scientists have hypothesized that vitamin B5 could somehow help our body better balance cortisol (stress hormone) and adapt to stress[293].

Vitamin B6 (Pyridoxine, pyridoxal, pyridoxamine, pyridoxal 5'-phosphate)
Source: Fish, organ meats, starchy vegetables like potatoes and non-citrus fruit.

Dose: 50-100mg

The active form of Vitamin B6 in the body is called pyridoxal 5' phosphate. It plays a role in over 100 enzyme reactions here. Vitamin B6 has been found to be lower in people with inflammatory health conditions[294].

Low levels of vitamin B6 have also been associated with depression in various medical studies[295]. So does this mean that a vitamin B6 deficiency could be causing the depression experienced in fibromyalgia? Unfortunately, scientists have not been able to answer this question yet. More research is still underway.

One possible theory could be that a B6 deficiency may be causing us to have low serotonin levels. Serotonin is our "happy hormone" which promotes a sense of well-being. Pyridoxal 5' phosphate (B6) is necessary in the production process of creating serotonin in our body[296]. Similarly, the production of GABA (the neurotransmitter that calms our brain/nervous system down) is also dependant on vitamin B6[297].

Vitamin B7 (Biotin)

Source: Eggs, cheese, organ meats, leafy greens, mushrooms, cauliflower, nuts, milk, grains and legumes.

Dose: 50mcg-100mcg+

You may have heard of Biotin (B7) by now, as it is highly marketed on social media as a supplement for thinning hair and nail growth. Biotin plays a role in the metabolism of fats and carbohydrates, as well as cell growth and energy production in the body[298]. Biotin is necessary for the production of a group of enzymes called carboxylases. Many of these biotin-dependant carboxylase enzymes are found in the mitochondria, where they play important roles in the production of ATP energy[299].

A recent study discovered a higher probability of biotin deficiency exists among fibromyalgia syndrome suffers; noting that B7 supplementation may be a useful therapy tool[300]. Furthermore, biotin may also help to rebuild and heal damaged nerve fibers in the body[301].

Vitamin B9 (Folate, Folic Acid, Folacin, 5-MTHF)
Source: kale and other dark green leafy vegetables, fruits, nuts, peas, beans, eggs, milk, cheese and grains.
Dose: 0.4 mg (400mcg)-5mg (pregnancy)
Vitamin B9 (Folic Acid) is important to the development of new cells. It is often prescribed in higher doses during pregnancy[302]. Additionally, pregnant women are frequently told to consume lots of whole foods. An emphasis is placed on the consumption of dark green leafy vegetables, as a way to naturally increase their folic acid intake.
In the body, folate is converted to 5-methyltetrahydrofolate (5-MTHF) which is the activated form of vitamin B9. This vitamin works to make red blood cells with the help of vitamin B12. Vitamin B9 also plays a role in regenerating a molecule called BH4 (tetrahydrobiopterin) in the body[303]. BH4 plays a key role in the creation of neurotransmitters like serotonin and dopamine.
When fibromyalgia syndrome and chronic fatigue subjects were given folic acid (B9) and vitamin B12, an overall improvement to fibromyalgia symptoms was seen over time[304].

Vitamin B12 (methylcobalamin, cyanocobalamin)
Source: Beef, chicken, liver, fish, dairy products including eggs.
Dose: 1mg (1000mcg)-100mg
As you may have already noticed, there are limited plant sources of vitamin B12. Years ago, I would hear my vegan friends rave about Brewer's Yeast or what is known as Nutritional Yeast. This yeast supposedly had lots of B12 in it. I later found out at my local grocery store that although nutritional yeast did in fact contain B vitamins, it did not have any B12 content. Luckily, there are many fortified nutritional yeasts and cereals on the market now; these have B12 added to them for individuals who do not eat meat.

When discussing B12 deficiency, also known as pernicious anemia, many factors come into play. First of all, B12 does not absorb easily into our gut, like the other water soluble B-vitamins do. Instead, B12 absorption is dependent on a substance called "intrinsic factor". Intrinsic factor is produced in the stomach, where it allows us to break down vitamin B12 from food and absorb it into our intestines[305]. So even if you are eating 10 steaks a day, without intrinsic factor you cannot absorb any vitamin B12. Our intrinsic factor levels will decrease as we age. Also, some people may not absorb B12 because they have antibodies which attack the intrinsic factor being produced in the stomach[306]. Finally, others may have stomach issues, being unable to maintain the proper stomach acid levels needed for intrinsic factor to be made[307]. To bypass the need for intrinsic factor, many doctors will prescribe B12 in the form of an injection or sublingual tablets. Sublingual B12 dissolves under the tongue; this allows the B12 to enter our blood stream through the tiny blood vessels there, eliminating dependence on the gut for B12 absorption.

Some of the symptoms of B12 deficiency include: dizziness with trouble walking; feeling weak and tired; numbness and tingling in the fingers and toes; difficulty thinking; memory loss; shortness of breath; and even constipation or diarrhea. Sound familiar? Yes, there are certainly many symptoms here which overlap with those experienced throughout fibromyalgia syndrome.

When studying women with fibromyalgia syndrome, researchers found low B12 levels in their spinal fluid, which they related to patient chronic fatigue[308].

Earlier we discussed a substance called SAMe (S-Adenosylmethionine) which is naturally produced by the body. SAMe supplements may act to better mitochondria functioning. Remember, the mitochondria are the power houses in our cells where ATP energy is produced. Vitamin B12 plays a role in the creation of the amino acid methionine, which is the major component of SAMe[309]. Hence, B12 is important to SAMe production.

SAMe has also been found to play a role in brain development.

Perhaps this is why B12 deficiency in elderly patients has been linked to brain wasting, dementia and Alzheimer's disease[310]. As a fibromyalgia patient who often experienced "fibro fog" and memory issues during flare-ups, I find this connection very interesting.

Vitamin B12 may also help with pain and poor sleep. In one large clinical study 1,149 patients with pain were given a B-complex of thiamine (B1), pyridoxine (B6) and cyanocobalmin (B12); 69% of them experienced symptom improvement within three weeks, with decreases in pain intensity, muscle weakness and numbness/tingling sensations[311]. Researchers also found that the B12 form called methylcobalmin improved sleep quality and decreased morning fatigue among some patients[312].

One key aspect to obtaining vital vitamins is gut health. If our digestive tract is unhealthy it will be harder to break down food and absorb these nutrients. The following chapter will discuss digestion and diet.

THE GUT HEALTH GUIDE

In earlier chapters we discussed the prevalence of digestive issues, like irritable bowel syndrome (IBS) in fibromyalgia. In my case, this consisted of painful bloating with periods of constipation followed by diarrhea. Everything I ate would make me feel a spasm-like pain in my gut. So in addition to feeling sore, moody and tired, I also had a bloated stomach that made me look flabby and overweight.

The reasons why fibromyalgia and IBS occur so commonly together is not well understood. However, many researchers believe that they are connected through what is known as the "brain-gut axis". This "axis" or pathway in the body is where the gut is believed to communicate with the brain, through biochemical signalling[313].

Isn't that profound?! Our gastrointestinal tract can communicate with our brain. There is more and more evidence coming through the scientific community to support the idea that the bacteria that naturally live in our digestive tract, our gut, and our brain, all communicate with each other through various neurotransmitters, hormones and signalling molecules[314]. Researchers have further emphasized this brain-gut connection through experimentation with gut bacteria. In one recent study, they found giving patients good gut bacteria (probiotics) decreased anxiety, worry and panic[315]. I mean come on! The potential for us to be able to alter our psychiatry by altering our gut health is amazing[316]. Could bettering our gastrointestinal health, help with pain and fatigue too?

Well, it is theorized that in some IBS cases the brain-gut axis is dysfunctional which messes up signalling to the brain; this in turn causes the increased pain responses of fibromyalgia syndrome[317]. We will discuss different approaches to fixing this dysfunction below.

Probiotics (Various Bacteria and certain types of yeast)
Source: Bacterial fermentation for supplements. Fermented Foods: Yogurt, Kefir, Sauerkraut, Kimchi, Tempeh, Kombucha, Pickles, Miso etc.
Dose: 25 Million CFUs - 20+ billion CFUs (varies based on age and disease state).
Probiotics are alive! They are bacteria which we can consume to help restore the balance of our own intestinal bacteria. Think of your gut as a beautiful forest. We have the actual gastrointestinal tract, which is the muscular and moist forest floor; this floor also has grass-like extensions that grow out of it and offer the "ground" (gut) protection. Amidst the grass and throughout the forest there are white flower patches, these represent our immune cells. In this forest we also have colonies of yeast and bacteria that live in harmony, for the most part. Sometimes, there can be an overgrowth of yeast, bad bacterial bugs and even parasites. The good bacteria our body naturally produces from digesting foods can keep these bad bugs at bay, allowing the "forest" to thrive.

From our mouth to our anus there is an intricate ecosystem that exists to provide us with everything from defences (immune system) to nutrients (digestion). Keeping this delicate system in balance is a critical key to health. When there is a lot of stress, antibiotic use, a poor diet and disease in our lives, our gut health may become compromised causing dysbiosis.

Dysbiosis is the term used for poor gut health that is caused by an imbalance of good bacteria versus bad bacteria and yeast. It has been linked to many health conditions. Dysbiosis is quite prevalent among fibromyalgia patients[318]. This makes sense based on our discussion above, the bacteria in the gut may alter functioning of the brain.

In one study where patients received probiotic supplements for 8 weeks; an increased quality life was reported by fibromyalgia patients[319]. The probiotic bacteria strains known as Bifidobacterium infantis and Lactobacillus casei were found to reduce inflammation and anxiety among chronic fatigue syndrome patients[320]. Although there is limited research on hormone level irregularities caused by dysbiosis in fibromyalgia syndrome, certain bacteria present in the gut have already been linked to the production of certain hormones in the brain[321].

Should we wait for more research then? What if we leave the dysbiosis untreated?

I've learned that this is not a good idea. Beyond the fact that bacteria in the gut have been shown to influence hormones and neurotransmitters in our body, not rebalancing dysbiosis may worsen health. Firstly, the bad bacteria may overgrow in the intestine; this could over stimulate our immune system making us sick and inflamed[322]. Secondly, this imbalance of gut bacteria may potentially cause a lowered intestinal permeability.

Intestinal permeability problems happen when the gut cannot regulate what materials pass through the intestines and enter our bodies' cells. Think of that forest floor, or gut, as a barrier where the "grass", "flowers" and good bacteria all act to keep bad stuff out. When the gut faces inflammation, stress, toxins and bacterial imbalances, the passages to the body from the gut can become more permeable or leaky[323].

At this point you may be wondering: Which probiotic should I take? Unless we examine every single food you eat and take poo samples to complete some expensive fecal testing, this question will be hard to answer. It is difficult to guess what good bacteria are missing from our individual systems. In order to ensure we replenish the gut appropriately, a broad-spectrum probiotic supplement can be taken. These globally available broad-spectrum probiotic supplements contain a range of different strains of helpful bacteria. For example, some supplements will offer 8 to 10 different types of bacteria including: Lactobacillus acidophilus, Lactobacillus rhamnosus, Lactobacillus plantarum, Bifidobacterium bifidum, Bifidobacterium longum and Lactobacillus casei.

Dosing for probiotic supplements will vary from patient to patient. Individuals who eat fermented foods will also get probiotics through this intake. As a general rule, scientists suggest about 1 billion probiotic microorganisms should be eaten daily[324]. However, in my clinical experience, the therapeutic dose for treating dysbiosis in adults is somewhere closer to 30 billion CFUs (colony forming units) of probiotics a day.

Probiotics can stimulate your immune system. So patients who are immune compromised, such as young children and HIV patients, may react poorly and be burdened by the high levels of bacteria in probiotics. A typical probiotic dose for a kid above 7 years of age would be only 25 million CFUs per day.

Ultimately, our diet determines which bacteria will be present in our gut[325]. A diet limited in chemically laced, processed foods and rich in a variety of whole foods will support the beneficial bacteria inside us.

<u>L-glutamine (Various Bacteria and certain types of yeast)</u>
<u>Source</u>: Chicken, fish, cabbage, lentils, beans, spinach and tofu. Naturally made by the body. Supplement pharmaceutical grade lab produced.
<u>Dose</u>: 750mg-5000mg (5g).

L-glutamine is an amino acid our body can usually make on its own. However, physical stressors like exercise and illness can create a higher demand for L-glutamine. Then we must obtain it from our diet and/or supplements.

L-glutamine is used by the body to produce an antioxidant called glutathione which helps protect our cells during stress[326]. L-glutamine also fuels the production of human growth hormone[327]. This hormone is important for muscle growth and cellular health.

In the gut, L-glutamine provides energy and protection to the intestinal cells[328]. Think of L-glutamine as a heavy snow fall in the "forest" (the gut). It comes in and covers everything. While protecting the "ground" and "grass", it also provides them with nutrients. L-glutamine acts like a thick, slimy, protective, mucilaginous barrier in the gut; giving the intestinal cells energy to heal, grow and function[329]. L-glutamine accomplishes this by stopping bad things (bacteria, viruses, parasites and undigested particles) from moving through the intestinal cells and into the bloodstream[330].

Situations of stress, allergies, antibiotics, poor nutrition, surgery and even alcoholism could cause our gut to become leaky, allowing toxins to enter. This "leaky gut" or increased intestinal permeability has been linked to many different gut disorders. A leaky gut may result in inflammation and irregular immune responses in the body[331].

In one experiment, scientists gave abdominal surgery patients 30g of L-glutamine supplements for 7 days after surgery[332]. They found the L-glutamine created a protective barrier in the intestines and stopped bacteria from getting into the gut. This decreased inflammation in the patients. Similarly, L-glutamine was found to decrease intestinal permeability in critically ill patients, and as a result reduced the frequency of infections they experienced[333]. This barrier function of L-glutamine sheds light on its protective potential for treating a range of gut issues including IBS[334].

L-glutamine supplements can be taken in capsule or powder form. During periods of stress and fibromyalgia-linked IBS flare ups, I will take 5g of L-glutamine powder in water each morning on an empty stomach.

Digestive Enzymes
Source: Animals (amylase, protease and lipase) and Plants (bromelain and papain).
Dose: Amylase 20,000 USP Units, Protease 20,000 USP Units,

Lipase 1,600 USP Units. Bromelain (250mg-1000mg), Papain (250mg-500mg).

Many of us experience problems digesting our food. Digestive enzymes can be taken to assist us in breaking down the fats, carbohydrates and proteins we consume in our diet. There are many different types of these enzymes available on the market. Most of them are sourced from animals such as the ox and pig. A simple blood test by your doctor can determine if you are low in any of your digestive enzymes. However, new research is underway regarding the benefits of digestive enzyme use among people who don't actually have enzyme deficiencies, yet still suffer from poor digestion/gut health[335].

Many of the digestive enzymes naturally made by our body are produced by the pancreas. Hence, these digestive enzymes are often referred to as pancreatic enzymes. These include Amylase, which breaks down sugars; Protease, which breaks down protein; and Lipase, which breaks down fats[336]. There is another digestive enzyme produced by our gut called lactase. This enzyme acts to break down a sugar called lactose, found in milk. The amount of enzymes produced by the pancreas has been shown to decrease by 44% in the elderly[337].

When being prescribed pancreatic enzymes by your doctor, you may notice the dosing is measured in United States Pharmacopeia Units (USP). This is a unit used in the US to measure a drug based on its weight and clinical effect. Internationally, digestive enzyme dosing could be measured in International Units (IU). For example, European scientists found that it takes 25,000 to 40,000 IUs of lipase to digest a meal, whereas much less of an amount is needed by the body to digest a snack[338].

Okay, so let's say your pancreas works fine but you still experience gas and bloating after each meal. Also, lots of undigested food can be seen in your stool. Does this warrant taking animal produced digestive enzymes?

For some patients, the answer to this question is yes. However, one controversial theory arises from this: Will supplementing with animal enzymes cause our body to naturally produce even less of our own enzymes in the long run? I mean why should the pancreas work to make what is already being supplemented?! Currently, there is no scientific research to substantiate this theory. Luckily, there are plant-based digestive enzymes available. These are found naturally in fruit.

Papain from papaya is a digestive enzyme that helps our gut break down proteins[339]. It can be consumed in a powdered supplement form and easily obtained by eating raw papaya. This protease is such a great aid in protein digestion that it is often added to commercial meat tenderizers. Papain is super cool. Besides the fact that it comes from the papaya fruit, it also exhibits anti-inflammatory, antioxidant and antimicrobial activity[340]. Yup, scientists have found that the digestive enzyme Papain fights against bad organisms in our body, such as E. coli, Salmonella and Staphylococcus[341].

Another plant-derived digestive enzyme is called Bromelain. This enzyme has been shown to assist in protein digestion and act as an anti-inflammatory[342]. Bromelain comes from pineapple. Higher concentrated amounts of Bromelain are actually found in the stem of the fruit[343].
Bromelain is a great supplement to explore when looking for natural digestion support. Firstly, researchers have found it is absorbed well when taken orally and maintains its protein breakdown activity in the gut. Secondly, it is cheaper to buy as a supplement because the stems of pineapple are often considered a food waste product. Finally, Bromelain is considered safe, even at doses of 12g a day[344].

There are a lot of opinions within the medical community regarding when digestive enzymes should be taken. A recent experiment finally laid this debate to rest. Scientists gave pancreatic enzymes to patients before, during or after their meal; they found digestion was better when the enzymes were taken with the food or after eating[345]. Based on this, I will often eat raw papaya and pineapple with my dinner or for dessert.

A FIBROMYALGIA DIET

Scientists have not yet established a standard diet for treating fibromyalgia. However, studies have shown a link between obesity and fibromyalgia[346]. Inflammation pathways in the body have also been linked to the development of fibromyalgia[347]. Therefore, focusing on an anti-inflammatory and weight loss diet (one that is lean, green and free of processed foods chalked full of chemicals) is a key approach for fibromyalgia patients. In the following section we will discuss the research that is shaping our diet protocol. I will also present sample meal plans to you.

Water

Before we get into that, let's talk about the most important dietary intervention of all: Water. It has been deemed our most important nutrient. Water is critical to the functioning of our body and without it we could die in as little as a few days[348]. Consuming water has even been found to help us with weight loss[349]. Not drinking enough water can lead to dehydration. This has been found to create negative mood changes[350], fatigue, headaches and dizziness[351]. As fibromyalgia sufferers, we especially want to avoid dehydration because it can cause muscle cramps, soreness and weakness[352].

When hydrating, drinking water is actually only about 70% to 80% of what our body gets each day. Generally, our body will get the remaining 30% to 40% of water from solid foods we eat[353]. Think of a fresh, juicy red apple. Over 80% of it is made up of water, which we intake as we eat it.

So, how much water should we drink each day?
This amount will depend from person to person.
Why?

The amount of water our body needs to function at optimum levels depends on many factors. When figuring this out for yourself there are a few questions you can ask. Firstly, what is your dietary intake in terms of water-rich fruits and vegetables? Secondly, do you exercise and lose water through sweat daily? Thirdly, what age are you and how much do you weigh? Finally, what is your environment like? Do you live in a hot and dry climate like the desert? All these things can affect our hydration needs[354].

There are a few math equations available to calculate how much water we need as individuals. However, because of all the varying factors listed above, I don't like to use these calculations. Our needs may change from day to day! One helpful trick is to make sure your pee is the colour of champagne. This is a healthy straw-like yellow. When urine is a concentrated dark yellow colour it can indicate dehydration. Alternatively, when our pee is completely clear in colour, this may indicate over hydration and too much water intake.

One popular water intake equation is your weight in pounds divided by the number 2. This number would give us the amount of water we need per day in ounces. For example, a sedentary, 200 pound person would need 100oz (12.5 cups) of water per day. In comparison, German researchers have found that there are no health benefits (other than preventing kidney stones) for men who drink more than 12 cups and women who drink more than 8.8 cups of water a day[355]. So drinking 8-12 cups a day is recommended and deemed adequate. We must remember that these amounts are for individuals who are sedentary and not burning calories, boosting metabolism and losing water in the form of sweat through exercise. As a result, The American College of Sports Medicine has recommended that for every 30 minutes of exercise we should add 12oz (1.5 cups) of water to our daily diet[356].

One brilliant way of getting nutrients, while ensuring we stay hydrated is through a diet rich in fruits and vegetables.

DIETARY CONSIDERATIONS

From very early childhood, we are encouraged to eat more fruits and vegetables. Not only do they provide our body with dietary fiber, but plenty of minerals and vitamins to fuel energy production too. Think about the wide array of colours found among fruits and vegetables. From red to green, to purple and orange, these foods get their colours from different phytochemicals. These are naturally occurring substances found in fruits and veggies. Beyond pigmentation, phytochemicals provide antioxidants that help protect our cells from damage and inflammation[357]. So many different phytochemicals have been identified. I believe that there may be even more found in fruits and vegetables, that scientists are yet to discover. As a simple way of obtaining different phytochemicals in our diet, I like to tell my patients to eat at least 5 different colours of fruits and vegetables a day.

Fruit and vegetables are the foundation of most fibromyalgia diet plans. Various diets for treating fibromyalgia have been proposed within the medical community. These include a vegan diet, gluten-free diet, FODMAP diet, low-calorie diet and a MSG/aspartame free diet[358].

THE VEGAN DIET

A vegan diet is rich in fruit, vegetables, beans and legumes. It is a diet that does not contain any food of animal origin. This means no eggs, no meat, no milk, no cheese etc. Some very strict vegans will also eliminate honey from their diet, as it is a bee product. When fibro researchers put patients on a vegan diet, they noticed a decrease in fibromyalgia symptoms within 3 months[359].

Similar results were found for fibromyalgia patients on a raw vegan diet. This is similar to a vegan diet that excludes all animal products. However, in a raw vegan diet, all foods are eaten raw or slowly dehydrated as opposed to cooked. As discussed earlier in this book, cooking can leach vitamins from our foods. Fibromyalgia patients on a raw vegan diet found they had increased vitality, with better physical, mental and emotional functioning within 4-7 months[360]. Who knew raw vegetables could change our mental and emotional health states too?

Another variation of the vegan diet is called the lacto-vegetarian diet. This diet is similar to a vegan diet as meat and eggs are absent; but lacto-vegetarians will eat dairy products such as milk, cheese and yogurt. After 4 weeks of doing core exercises and eating a lacto-vegetarian diet, fibromyalgia patients experienced decreased pain and body fat loss[361].

THE MEDITERRANEAN DIET

Another diet, sometimes prescribed to fibromyalgia patients is the Mediterranean diet. This diet is heavily plant-based with a focus on vegetables and fruits. Chicken is only consumed once a week. Red meat, like beef or lamb could be consumed once a week to once a month. This diet is void of butter and has healthy fats like olive oil and nuts added to it instead. There are a lot of herbs used in the Mediterranean diet; these replace salt. Turmeric and ginger are often added to foods for their anti-inflammatory properties and flavour. In the daily Mediterranean diet you will see some dairy (milk, cheese and yogurt), beans, legumes and whole grain breads. The main source of protein and fats in this diet comes from the abundant amount of fish and seafood eaten.

Eating a Mediterranean diet has been shown to decrease inflammation in the body[362]. This makes sense because it is low in red meat and processed foods, while being high in omega-3 fats. Also, this diet is often rich in turmeric and ginger which are natural anti-inflammatory seasonings.

Research has found that the Mediterranean diet helps to prevent bone loss (osteoporosis) in women suffering from fibromyalgia syndrome[363].

The omega-3 fats in the Mediterranean diet are mainly from fish. When fibromyalgia patients eat omega-3 rich fish 2 to 5 times a week, and fruits and vegetables every day, they experience lower levels of depression[364]. Drinking sugary drinks and eating processed meats (like cured ham) may lead to low mood among women suffering from fibromyalgia.

You may be wondering: What the hell is wrong with eating lots of red meat?

Red meat is high in a different kind of fat. This saturated fat is bad for us when compared to the omega-3 fats which are healthy. In a recent experiment, scientists were able to create fibromyalgia-like pain in mice by feeding them a high saturated fat diet[365]. Hence, all those steaks and lamb chops in our Western diet could potentially be making fibromyalgia pain worse.
As a general rule, when eating animal protein, try to consume the ones which have fewer legs. Fish have no legs and will be at the top of our desired food list. Second, will be lean chicken and turkey, they have only 2 legs. Finally, we must try to limit the four legged foods: cows, pigs, lamb, goat etc.

When examining all of these potential fibromyalgia diets, I want you to ask yourself which one works best for you. Can you stick to this diet and make it a permanent lifestyle change? Our main goal is consistency. It is no easy feat going vegan. I can attest to this, as I've been an on again/off again vegan for many years. Dietary restrictions can be stressful and are a huge part of many fibromyalgia protocols.
On the one hand, we do need to watch what we eat in order to sustain energy, keep weight down and avoid fibromyalgic flare-ups. On the other hand, we also need to be happy and live! It's stressful having to restrict and eliminate things from your diet. When people say this is just the reality of having a chronic disease, they actually have a valid point. However, we need to be kind to ourselves and find a balance with a fibromyalgia diet and lifestyle plan that is realistic and easy to adapt to. For me, the Mediterranean diet worked best long-term.

THE LOW FODMAP DIET

For the fibromyalgia patients who also suffer from severe IBS, the low FODMAP diet may be a better choice. Low FODMAP diet stands for the following: low Fermentable Oligo-Di-Mono-saccharides And Polyols diet. These are fancy names for small carbohydrates found in certain foods which have been found to cause gut pain, diarrhea, bloating and gas in people with IBS[366]. In the low FODMAP diet, eliminating these foods (high FODMAP foods) is a key to stopping the digestive discomfort. An example of some of the foods eliminated are garlic and onions; milk and yogurt; mangoes; honey; blackberries; asparagus, and cauliflower. Subsequently, scientists wanted to test this diet out on fibromyalgia patients. During a 2 month study they found fibromyalgia patients who followed a low FODMAP plan had a decrease in waist size and muscle pain[367].

This further highlights how a properly, tailored diet may lessen our suffering throughout fibromyalgia syndrome.

A FIBROMYALGIA DIET PLAN

I will present to you examples of a typical diet plan for an omnivorous and active fibromyalgia patient. It is important to try your best to ensure the fruits, vegetables, eggs, dairy and meat in this meal plan are pesticide, hormone-free and organic. You can make these options your own by adding herbs, spices and citrus to your liking. Adding ginger and turmeric to as many meals as possible is also recommended. Oils used to prepare these meals include: Grapeseed oil, Avocado oil, Coconut oil, Canola oil and uncooked, cold pressed, extra-virgin olive oil for the salads. You can also add more or less food into this plan based on your dietary needs, taste preferences, and weight loss goals.

Monday

Breakfast: 1/3 cup cooked Oatmeal + 1 sliced banana + 1 teaspoon cinnamon + 1tbsp flax oil. You can sweeten this with a natural sweetener like stevia or monk fruit.

Mid-morning Snack: 1 small apple with 3 thin slices of skim mozzarella cheese.

Lunch: 4oz grilled chicken breast + 3 cups of cooked or raw dark green salad (spinach, rapini or kale) + cold pressed extra virgin olive oil and balsamic dressing.

Mid-afternoon snack: 10 brown rice crackers with ½ an avocado mashed (season to taste).

Dinner: 1 steak extra lean (pan grilled) + 10 stalks of steamed or sautéed asparagus + 1/3 cup of ricotta cheese.

Evening Snack (optional): 7-10 raw almonds.

Tuesday
Breakfast: 2 hardboiled eggs.

Mid-morning Snack: 1 plain rice cake with natural peanut butter (no sugar added) and 1/2 sliced banana on top.

Lunch: Homemade lean ground chicken or turkey meatballs (meat and seasoning only no breadcrumbs added) + 3 cups of dark green salad + olive oil dressing + 1 cup of steamed broccoli.

Mid-afternoon snack: 1 fresh peach.

Dinner: Wildcaught Salmon (if frozen or fresh is not available then canned will suffice) + salad of choice. The salad must include at least 3 vegetables.

Evening Snack (optional): 1-2 cups of raw vegetables + 2 tablespoons of hummus or greek yogurt for dipping.

Wednesday

Breakfast: 1/3 cup of cottage cheese with ½ cup blueberries, 5 strawberries sliced, 2 tablespoons chia seeds, 1 teaspoon cinnamon and ½ cup raw almonds or walnuts on top.

Mid-morning Snack: 1 pear with $1/3^{rd}$ cup of raw walnuts.

Lunch: 4oz of baked cod fish (season with dill, olive oil and garlic) + 2 cups sautéed greens or a fresh salad of choice.

Mid-afternoon snack: 1/2 to 1 whole cucumber sliced up + 5 baby carrots + 10 cherry tomatoes.

Dinner: 2-3 cups beans (fresh or canned) sautéed with onions, peppers, mushrooms and herbs.

Evening Snack (optional): 1 rice cake with natural nut or seed butter on top (peanut, almond or sesame for example).

Thursday

Breakfast: 1 whole egg + ½ cup egg whites scrambled. Add in a handful of vegetables when cooking for a scrambled frittata. (1/2 onion, tomatoes, herbs, green pepper or even frozen vegetables).

Mid-morning Snack: 1 small sized orange or tangerine. 2 squares of 70% dark chocolate.

Lunch: 4oz grilled chicken breast + 3 cups dark green salad + olive oil/balsamic dressing.

Mid-afternoon snack: 1-2 cups raw vegetables of choice + 2 tablespoons of hummus.

Dinner: 2 cups of steamed cauliflower + 8 lean turkey or chicken meatballs on top. Mash and the steamed cauliflower like you would to make mashed potatoes.

Evening Snack (optional): 5 brown rice crackers and ½ a mashed avocado.

Friday

Breakfast: 1/3 cup cooked oatmeal + 1tbsp flax oil + 1/2 cup blueberries + 10 raw walnuts. You can add 1 tsp real maple syrup and a pinch cinnamon to flavour. Use almond milk instead of water to make you oatmeal creamy.

Mid-morning Snack: 1 small apple + 5 raw almonds + 1 slice of skim mozzarella cheese.

Lunch: 3 cups of Vegetable soup.
You can make this by boiling chopped fresh and/or frozen vegetables covered in a pot with some vegetable or chicken stock. Once the veggies are soft and the soup has cooled-blend the mixture with an immersion blender until it reaches a thick and smooth consistency. You can also leave this soup chunky. One combo I enjoy includes: 4 cups of organic vegetable stock, 1 cup of water, ½ a cauliflower, 2 small potatoes, 3 red peppers, 3 car-

rots, 1 chopped zucchini, 1 onion, 3 cloves of garlic, ½ cup of green peas, 5 stalks of celery, 1 head of broccoli, basil and coriander.

Mid-afternoon snack: 1 rice cracker with organic nut butter with some sliced banana and chia seeds on top. You can also sprinkle some cinnamon on top of this.

Dinner: Asian stir-fry with any lean protein (chicken, fish, tofu or beans) of choice. Add snow peas, bokchoy, mushrooms, broccoli, carrots, onions or any vegetables you like to this stirfry. Use a low sodium soy sauce or tamari sauce when seasoning. Don't forget the ginger and turmeric! You can eat this stir-fry with 1/2 cup of quinoa or brown rice.

Evening Snack (optional): 1/2 cup of mixed berries: blueberries, blackberries, strawberries, raspberries + 5-10 raw almonds.

Saturday
Breakfast: 2 protein pancakes topped with 1/2 cup mixed berries and 5 crushed walnuts. You can add 1tsp of pure maple syrup or sprinkle some monkfruit or stevia powder on top to sweeten the pancakes. Other toppings options include: greek yogurt, sunflower, hemp or pumkin seeds, shredded coconut, natural peanut butter etc.

How to make protein pancakes

Ingredients:
2 scoops of high quality vegan protein powder
1/2 banana (optional)
2 egg whites
1-2 teaspoon raw organic cacao powder
1 teaspoon cinnamon
2+ tablespoons cold water
1-2 teaspoons Cold Pressed Organic Coconut Oil for cooking the protein pancake

Place protein powder, banana, egg whites, cacao and cinnamon in a mixing bowl or blender. Whisk or blend the mixture until a smooth batter forms. Add cold water, 1 tablespoon at a time to help you achieve a pancake batter consistency. Place the coconut oil in a non-stick pan. Heat the pan to medium-low on the stove top. Add in the pancake batter. Allow one side to cook (you will see small bubbles emerging to the top). Once cooked, flip the pancake and cook other side. Your pancake should flip like a regular one. Cooking this at a low temperature is the key to keeping this pancake formed and stopping it from breaking apart or scrambling up in the pan.

Mid-morning Snack: 1 rice cracker with 1/2 avocado mashed on top. This can be seasoned with some garlic powder, sesame seeds and salt and pepper.

Lunch: Green salad of choice with 1 can of tuna. You can season the tuna to preference and add in some fresh lemon, organic corn and celery to your salad. Fresh herbs like parsley, dill and coriander will also brighten up this meal.

Mid-afternoon snack: 1 sliced cucumber topped with some Greek yogurt.

Dinner: 4oz grilled chicken breast with 1/2 cup sautéed squash, onions, broccoli and asparagus. You can also prepare a mixed bean salad (fresh or canned) seasoned with some olive oil, salt, pepper and herbs. 1/2 the bean salad can be added to the meal.

Evening Snack (optional): 1 small purple plum + 7 raw almonds.

Sunday
Breakfast: 2 protein pancakes topped with 1/2 banana, 1 tsp pure maple syrup (or stevia) and 2 tablespoons unsweetened coconut flakes.

Mid-morning Snack: 1 nectarine

Lunch: Grilled shrimp skewers (10 shrimp) with a dark green salad and 2 roasted or grilled zucchini.

<u>Mid-afternoon snack</u>: 2 medium tomatoes sliced with 4 slices of fresh mozzarella. Season this with olive oil, basil, salt and pepper. You can eat this like a salad or with 5 brown rice crackers.

<u>Dinner</u>: 4oz broiled Pacific salmon with lots of lightly sautéed broccoli + garlic + olive oil + 1 small dark green salad and an olive oil/balsamic dressing.

<u>Evening Snack (optional)</u>: Homemade "Ice cream": Blend 1 frozen organic banana, 1 tsp cacao and add a few sliced almonds on top. You can also add in 1 teaspoon of coconut oil to this frosty dessert.

<u>Week 2</u>
<u>Monday</u>
<u>Breakfast</u>: 1L Green Spinach Smoothie. To make, blend: 5-8 small chunks of frozen mango + 1/2-1 cup fresh organic spinach + 1/2 thumb-sized piece of peeled fresh ginger root + 1/2-1 teaspoon turmeric powder + 1/2 teaspoon cinnamon powder + 1/2 tsp spirulina powder (optional) + 1 litre filtered water.. This drink actually tastes really good! Somehow the frozen mangoes and ginger cancel out the taste of the spinach.

<u>Mid-morning Snack:</u> 1 rice cake with 1 tablespoon raw organic almond butter on top.

<u>Lunch</u>: 2 oz broiled chicken breast + basil pesto sauce + 2 cups steamed broccoli + 1/3 cup brown rice pasta.

<u>Mid-afternoon snack</u>: 10 raw almonds.

<u>Dinner</u>: Baked white fish (Sole, Cod or wild caught Tilapia) + lemon and dill dressing + 8 stalks steamed asparagus + ½ cup sautéed mushrooms. On the side: a small green salad + olive oil dressing.

<u>Evening Snack (optional)</u>: 1 pomegranate or 1/2 cup berries with some stevia on top.

Tuesday
Breakfast: 2 boiled eggs.

Mid-morning Snack: 1 apple sliced and topped with 1 table-spoon of peanut butter + 1 tablespoon of chia seeds.

Lunch: 2-3 cups homemade vegetable soup.

Mid-afternoon snack: 10 raw almonds and 1/2 avocado sliced.

Dinner: 1/2 cup organic ground beef sautéed with green vegetables and tomatoes, served on top of one cup zucchini noodles. You can purchase a hand-held vegetable spiralizer to make the zucchini noodles spaghetti thin or you can use a standard peeler for thicker noodles.

Evening Snack (optional): Raw vegetables, like broccoli, cauliflower and cucumber + 2 tablespoons of hummus for dipping. You can make your own low-fat hummus by blending cooked chickpeas (canned or freshly boiled) with some olive oil, salt, pepper and paprika.

Wednesday
Breakfast: 1 egg and 1/2 cup egg whites cooked into an omelette with onion, tomato, garlic and cilantro. Use 1 tsp coconut oil or grapeseed oil to cook this. Serve on top of 2 cups arugula.

Mid-morning Snack: 1 small orange with 2 squares of 70% dark chocolate.

Lunch: 1 cup bean salad + 1 cup dark greens (kale, rapini, spinach) with olive oil and balsamic dressing.

Mid-afternoon snack: 1 rice cake with 1/2 mashed avocado on top.

Dinner: 4oz grilled salmon. 3cups spinach + arugula salad + olive oil vinaigrette dressing + ½ cup steamed squash.

Evening Snack (optional): 1 cup vegetable soup.

Thursday
Breakfast: 1L Green Spinach Smoothie

Mid-morning Snack: 1 rice cake with 1 tablespoon of cashew or peanut butter on top.

Lunch: 2 boiled eggs + 3cups dark greens salad + olive oil dressing. You can also add in 1 cup of steamed broccoli to your salad.

Mid-afternoon snack: 1 apple with 3 thin slices of mozzarella cheese.

Dinner: 2 cups steamed cauliflower. Mash and season cauliflower like you would potatoes. Serve this with lean turkey or chicken meatballs on top.

Evening Snack (optional): 10 raw almonds and 2 Brazil nuts.

Friday
Breakfast: 1/3 cup cooked Oatmeal + 1 sliced banana + 1 teaspoon cinnamon + 1tbsp flax oil. You can sweeten this with a natural sweetener like stevia or monk fruit.

Mid-morning Snack: 1 apple with 10 raw almonds.

Lunch: 4oz grilled chicken breast with 3 cups of green salad of choice + 1 cup steamed cauliflower or Brussels sprouts.

Mid-afternoon snack: 5 brown rice crackers with 1/2 avocado mashed and seasoned to taste.

Dinner: 4oz broiled wild-caught, Pacific salmon with sautéed broccoli + garlic + olive oil + 1 cup dark green salad on the side.

Evening Snack (optional): Homemade "Ice cream": Blend 1 frozen organic banana, 1 tsp cacao and add a few sliced almonds on top.

Saturday

Breakfast: 1 L Green Spinach Smoothie.

Mid-morning Snack: 1 sliced apple topped with 1 tablespoon peanut butter, 1 tablespoon hemp heart seeds and a sprinkle of cinnamon.

Lunch: 2 cups steamed cauliflower. Mash and season cauliflower like you would potatoes. Serve this with 2 oz of grilled or baked white fish.

Mid-afternoon snack: 1/2 cup of mixed berries. You can sweeten this with a little stevia on top.

Dinner: Asian stirfry with any lean protein (chicken, fish, tofu or beans) and vegetables of choice. Serve with 1/2 cup of quinoa or brown rice.

Evening Snack (optional): Homemade "Ice cream": Blend 1 frozen organic banana, 1 tsp cacao and add a few sliced almonds on top.

Sunday
Breakfast: 2 protein pancakes.

Mid-morning Snack: 1 tangerine and 5-8 raw walnuts.

Lunch: 2 rice cakes or 2 thin slices of whole grain toast topped with avocado and egg salad. You can make this salad by chopping or smashing 1 avocado and 2 boiled eggs until they form a creamy or chunky mixture. Don't forget to season this with herbs and spices. You can also add chopped onion to the salad topping.

Mid-afternoon snack: raw vegetables and 3 tablespoons of hummus for dipping.

Dinner: 4 oz wild-caught salmon (baked or canned) with 3 cups green salad of choice.

Evening Snack (optional): 1/2 cup mixed berries + 5 chopped almonds on top.

MIND AND BODY WORK

Now that we have implemented an anti-inflammatory diet plan for ourselves, it is time for us to put in the mind and body work for healing fibromyalgia syndrome.

MIND

As discussed in-depth, the brain plays a major role in fibromyalgia. From stress to mood, to pain, it is an essential point of focus here.

Music Therapy

Do you ever notice that in real life and in the movies there is always relaxing music playing in spas? What about elevator music; what purpose does it serve?

Well, researchers have found that listening to music could actually decrease levels of both pain and stress in our daily lives[368]. In a study where fibromyalgia patients were given relaxing music to listen, scientists discovered they experienced lower tenderness and higher physical functioning[369]. Similar results were found when 60 fibromyalgia patients listened to music once every day for a month; they had a resultant lower pain and depression level[370].

Currently, there is a lot of music therapy research underway. One experiment has even provided evidence that showed singing may positively improve mood, stress and the immune systems of cancer patients[371]. This may come as no surprise to those of you who feel rejuvenated after a 10 minute concert, consisting of you singing in your shower.

Mindful Meditation

For decades, mindfulness meditation has been used as a tool to treat chronic pain[372]. To be mindful means to focus your mind on the present moment. Our minds are constantly running, to a point where our thoughts can become cluttered and busy with inconsequential things. Sometimes we are so focused on the past trauma, fibromyalgia pain, daily stressors, worrying about others and the things we need to get done that we forget to connect with our bodies. Mindfulness meditation challenges us to clear our mind, be in the moment and focus only on our breathing, our body, one chosen points of focus, or nothing at all.

Have you ever tried to meditate and channel all your attention on what you are experiencing in the present moment? Well, it sounds easier than done. There may be frequent nagging moments where your brain will drift off to worries of "I have to pick up the kids from school" and "What am I going to make for dinner?" These tangent thoughts of common stressors can lessen as you practice this form of meditation.

Many doctors will prescribe mindfulness meditation to their patients, as it has been found to decrease fibromyalgia pain and tender points[373]. Some believe that mindfulness-based meditation may work to alter physical, nerve and psychological pathways in our body[374]. Thus far, neurologists have found practising mindfulness meditation relieves stress by somehow affecting an area in the brain called the amygdala[375]. The amygdala plays a role in processing certain emotions, like fear for example. Despite the large amount of scientific studies supporting mindfulness meditation for fibromyalgia pain management, a lot of the specifics, such as how it affects our body, are still unknown[376]. What we do know is that this type of meditation can help people with social anxiety disorder control their emotions better[377] Mindfulness meditation may also help to decrease the symptoms of depression[378]. Isn't that amazing? By spending a few minutes each day focusing on our breathing, our body and being in the moment with our present sensations, we can clear the stressors in our minds. I really believe mindfulness meditation may present our body with a great opportunity to heal.

If you would like to implement meditation into your daily

life there are multiple resources on this topic available. These include books, instructional blogs and Youtube videos. Alternatively, many local mental health centers and hospitals offer mindfulness-based stress reduction programs. Often, mindfulness meditation can be taught by a licensed psychologist. My psychologist incorporated meditation into our biweekly sessions, in addition to a cognitive behavioural therapy plan that she devised for me during my fibromyalgia treatment.

Cognitive Behavioural Therapy
One common theme for many of us fibromyalgia sufferers is trauma. This could be physical (in my case a car accident) or unresolved hurt, fear and anger from some emotional trauma (such as a divorce or the death of a loved one).

Cognitive Behavioural Therapy (CBT) is a popular mental health therapy. CBT consists of talk therapy, journaling and other exercises which act to challenge our often distorted and irrational thoughts. If you are someone who has trouble coping with negative thought cycles and always thinks the worst will happen (catastrophizing), CBT may be of great use to you. Practicing CBT can provide us with an arsenal of techniques which we can use every time we feel stressed and overwhelmed. This technique works on the premise that if we are able to alter our destructive thought patterns to more positive and rational ones, then we may be able to behave in a more stress free way.

For fibromyalgia patients positive changes in physical functioning, pain and coping may occur in as little as 10-20 CBT sessions[379]. Researchers have found that the long-term effects of this therapy included reduced negativity, better mood, as well as less overall pain and disability among fibromyalgia sufferers[380]. In one experiment, 79 subjects with fibromyalgia syndrome took a meditation based, stress reduction CBT program. After less than 3 months of these weekly 2 hour CBT sessions, 67% of them had improved fibromyalgia symptoms[381].

There are many workbooks available on CBT. These emphasize weekly homework assignments and putting the learned CBT skills to work in daily life. Although it is suggested to seek assistance from a trained therapist, you can also learn and practice CBT skills through various self-learning tools. In fact, one study found that an online CBT program called MoodGYM helped fibromyalgia patients. This internet accessible, at-home CBT program was found to reduce tender point pain and benefitted fibromyalgia patients with depression and anxiety[382].

Breathing

When you think about one of the most painful human experiences, giving birth may come to mind. Some people have compared labour pain to 20 bones breaking at the same time. As a result of the pain, we often see pregnant women practicing breathing exercises to assist with the birthing process. Deep breathing exercises have been found to be very effective in reducing labour pain[383]. Similarly, studies have found that practicing breathing exercises decreases tender points and improves self-management of pain among fibromyalgia patients[384]. Many of the physical exercises prescribed to fibromyalgia patients contain breathing exercises as a component.

There are many types of breathing exercises. A simple way to start is to keep your body relaxed. Inhale slowly for a count of 5, through your nose. Then breathe out slowly for a count of 5, through your mouth. Make sure your jaw is relaxed as you exhale. Repeat this breathing exercise daily for several minutes and incorporate it into your exercise regimen.

Toxicity

Before we move on from the mind to treating our body, I want to discuss toxicity.

In our lives we will inevitably encounter toxic people, be exposed to toxic environments and partake in toxic habits. Toxic people are the worst. These are those coworkers, frenemies, family members, romantic partners and even well intentioned friends that surround us with negative energy. These individuals may drain us with their attitude and personal demands; they may cause us to doubt ourselves and partake in negative self talk; or even be outright abusive towards us.

In my opinion, a toxic environment is anywhere that I feel super stressed or unhappy. Vibes don't lie. Learning to trust my gut, when it comes to bad vibes, played a large role in my healing. This has allowed me to protect myself from people and situations that slowed down my healing process and aggravated my emotional and physical pain.

As for bad habits, in retrospect, none of them are really worth the worsening of fibromyalgia symptoms and the increased suffering.

If we're lucky, we will get an average of 88 years to live. This is all we have. Yes, we need to be kind to ourselves. Yes, we deserve to be pain-free and healthy. Yes, we should only surround ourselves with the people and places that make us feel supported and happy.

Toxic people, toxic environments and toxic habits: Get them the f*ck out of your life!

If you find this absolutely impossible to do, then find time to distance yourself from these stressors. Take time to recharge your batteries. Learn to say "NO" and prioritize yourself. Self-care is like the in-flight safety rule, where you must put on your oxygen mask first before helping others. If you run out of oxygen, you are of no service to anyone else!

BODY

The one thing none of us want to do when we're in pain is exercise. However, limiting our activity and leading sedentary lives, can cause weight gain, depression and worsen our fibromyalgia symptoms. During one of my fibro flare-ups, I sought the help of a seasoned rheumatologist. She told me that beyond pain medications and supplements, the most important prescription she could give me was exercise. "Get moving" she said, "Keep that blood flowing and your muscles will function properly." At that point, this seemed like the impossible to me. As a previous runner, weight lifter and sports enthusiast, fibromyalgia pain had taken away any motivation for exercise. This is where I learned how to "exercise to tolerance".

Exercising to tolerance is when we only do exercises that we are able to endure. No more killing ourselves at the gym and straining our body beyond what it is comfortable with. Tolerance to exercise is built by starting with low-impact exercises and moving towards the maximum work load our body can handle. In the earlier chapters of this book, we spoke about endorphins. Endorphins are released by our body during exercise[385]. This is important in fibromyalgia because endorphins interact with our opiate receptors in the brain, where they reduce our pain perception. Hence, exercise can positively change our pain experience. Exercise has a positive effect on cortisol levels and different pain receptors in the body; this makes the physical stress from exercise good for us in comparison to the bad stressors we encounter in our daily lives[386].

For fibromyalgia patients, 6 months of moderate, low-impact

exercise has been found to improve pain symptoms, mood and functioning[387]. Aerobic exercise has also been found to improve low energy and feelings of chronic fatigue[388]. Some common exercises for fibromyalgic patients include walking, swimming, yoga and Tai-chi.

Walking

Many doctors recommend walking to their fibromyalgia patients[389]. This form of aerobic exercise can get our heart rate and breathing up while still remaining low impact on our bodies. This may benefit fibromyalgia syndrome by strengthening muscles[390].

Swimming/Aquatic Exercise

I think of swimming as a fun activity I've enjoyed since childhood. Swimming can actually be a great way to get physically strong and burn calories. We are virtuously weightless in water. Gravity having less of an effect on us while in the water will take a lot of stress off of our body. This can allow us to increase flexibility and get our painful, stiff joints moving. In one experiment, fibromyalgia patients performed aerobic exercises in a pool for 1 hour, twice a week. After 8 months, they had less inflammation in their bodies; which was confirmed by the lowered levels of inflammatory markers in their blood work[391].

It is important to note that although swimming and aqua aerobics are beneficial cardio, they are not weight-bearing exercises. Weight bearing exercises benefit our bones because they force us to resist against gravity. These exercises could include walking or lifting free weights to tolerance. Researchers have found that a combination of both aerobic and weight bearing exercise is effective in reducing pain, depression and fatigue in people with fibromyalgia syndrome[392]. Another popular weight bearing exercise is yoga. Yoga consists of a lot of stretching, relaxation and breathing too. However, in yoga we will often use our own body weight to create resistance during certain poses.

Yoga

3000 years old, yoga is deemed as not only exercise for the body, but also the mind. Yoga can create a state of relaxation and peace among those who practice it. Physically, yoga promotes flexibility, strength and endurance. This form of exercise consists of breathing, self-awareness and movements that challenge our muscles.

The top reasons why fibromyalgia patients don't want to practice yoga is because they are worried the yoga poses will be too difficult, or that this type of stretching exercise will cause pain[393]. Both of these are misconceptions. Firstly, yoga is a type of exercise that can be adjusted in skill and intensity level, to your tolerance. Secondly, research has found that yoga actually helps people who suffer from chronic pain[394].

Fibromyalgia patients, who practiced yoga at home for 20 minutes per day, as well as attended one weekly yoga class, were found to have lower tender points and less overall muscle pain within 3 months[395]. These yoga classes consisted of a 20 minute meditation, 10 minutes of breathing exercises and 40 minutes of gentle stretching poses. In another 2 month experiment, women with fibromyalgia who practiced yoga had positive changes to body pain, stress hormone (cortistol) levels and mental functioning[396]. This potential of yoga to counteract the mental and physical disability in fibromyalgia syndrome makes it worth trying.

Tai Chi (Tai ji, Tai ji quan)

Tai ji quan also known as Tai Chi is a gentle martial arts exercise from China. It consists of slow body movements with meditation and deep breathing.

Researchers have found that practicing Tai Chi for 1 hour, twice a week, helps fibromyalgia sufferers with their pain, depression and sleep quality[397]. Furthermore, Tai Chi is a common exercise prescription in fibromyalgia syndrome because it improves balance and increases our physical functioning and mobility[398].

Qi Gong (Chi kun, Chi gung, Qigong)
Qigong is another ancient Chinese practice used for healing the body. This exercise is similar to Tai Chi, as it consists of body movements, meditation and mindfulness breathing. However, Qigong is less complex that Tai Chi; with more gentle, simple and slow movements. Despite this, Qigong is still very effective in treating chronic pain[399].

Fibromyalgia patients who practiced Qi gong for 30-45 minutes a day were found to have less pain, better sleep, and an overall improvement in mental and physical health[400].

Check your city's parks and recreation, local community center and gym for Tai Chi and Qigong classes. Additionally, there are many online resources which can assist you with at-home exercises.

EXERCISE PRESCRIPTION

A fibromyalgia exercise prescription will vary from person to person. It is important to stick to an individualized plan, based on your level of tolerance. We all have different levels of functioning and flare-ups; these can change drastically over the course of the disease. Beginning at a low intensity will prevent injury and ensure we stay motivated and consistent in our practice of mind-body exercises.

At this point you may be wondering: Do I have to work out every day? The answer to this is: it depends on you. Being sedentary is bad. Hence, exercising everyday is recommended for many individuals. However, scientists have found that in fibromyalgia syndrome, low to moderate intensity exercise, practiced even just 2-3 times a week is enough to decrease pain, improve mood and increase our quality of life[401].

PHYSICAL THERAPY

Exercise is a major form of physical therapy used to treat fibromyalgia. Other physical therapies that have been used in fibromyalgia include electric stimulation, massage therapy and acupuncture. A Physical Therapist, Naturopathic Doctor, Registered Massage Therapist or Chiropractor can provide some or all of these services to you.

Electric Stimulation
Let me introduce you all to my best friend, who numbs my muscle pain quickly: The TENS Machine. TENS stands for Transcutaneous Electrical Nerve Stimulation. A TENS machine will send an electric current into sticky patches placed on our skin. These sticky patches (which are also called electrodes) can be positioned over our areas of pain. The pattern and intensity of the electrical current or pulses can then be adjusted to our comfort level. TENS has shown potential benefit in decreasing the hypersensitive and heightened pain responses seen among fibromyalgia patients[402].

The TENS machine works by increasing the concentration of endorphins and opioid growth factors in our bloodstream; It also numbs pain by activating different sensory nerves and various pain receptors in the brain[403]. When fibromyalgia patients were treated with a TENS, they were found to be less hypersensitive and experienced lowered soreness and fatigue[404].

Electric stimulation has also been found to be effective when combined with acupuncture[405]. Electroacupuncture is when electrode clamps are attached to acupuncture needles. An electric current then travels through the needles into the muscles in which they are inserted. This allows your physician to enhance the stimulation of acupuncture points during treatment.

Currently, there are many hand-held TENS machines available on the market for home use. Most of these units are inexpensive. Many insurance companies will also cover the cost of a TENS unit if it is prescribed by your doctor. You can purchase a unit online or through your health care practitioner.

Massage Therapy

I have noticed huge differences in opinion among my fibromyalgia patients when it comes to massage therapy. Many of my patients are hesitant to try massage, due to the fact that any physical pressure on their body is painful and even intolerable during fibromyalgic flare-ups. Some other patients find the manipulation of their muscles, ligaments, tissues and joints through massage therapy, offers them temporary relief of fibromyalgic stiffness and pain. Scientific research has established that massage therapy can actually benefit fibromyalgia symptoms in the short-term[406]. It is well known within the medical community that massage therapy can reduce pain, anxiety and depression among patients undergoing cancer care[407]. Similarly, massage may improve mood, while providing better physical functioning and less muscle tension in those suffering from chronic pain[408]. It is best to seek an assessment by a Registered Massage Therapist (RMT) specializing in fibromyalgia pain prior to beginning any massage treatment program.

THE ACUPUNCTURE PROTOCOL

Acupuncture is an over 2000 year old form of Chinese medicine. It is used globally as an alternative therapy for many health disorders, from infertility to chronic pain. During acupuncture, a health care practitioner will insert thin needles through the skin into specifically selected points on the body. The length, depth and angle of the acupuncture needles will vary based on the area being treated and the points that are chosen. Acupuncture, in general does not hurt. Normal sensations you can expect once the needles are in, include burning, heaviness, warmth and tingling. There should not be sharp or shooting pain from the needles after insertion. The needles are often left in the body for 30-45 minutes. Many people find acupuncture relaxing and fall asleep during treatment. In North America, most government registered Traditional Chinese Medicine practitioners and Naturopathic Doctors will study and practice acupuncture for a minimum of 4 years, before becoming licensed to treat patients in their province or state.

It is common to see acupuncture as a physical therapy component in many fibromyalgia treatment protocols. After fibromyalgia patients received 20 sessions of acupuncture in one study, researchers found these subjects had lower tender points and pain[409]. These positive results also lasted for 3 months after the acupuncture treatments were stopped. Beyond pain, acupuncture sessions may also help those of us who experience "pins-and-needles" or numbness and tingling sensations due to nerve damage in our tissues[410]. Furthermore, it has been proposed that acupuncture may reduce stress, decrease anxiety[411] and maybe even fatigue[412] in some individuals. However, much more research is needed to fully establish Traditional Chinese Medicine (TCM) within the framework of modern science. This is why there are still some doctors who don't believe in the effectiveness of acupuncture. It is an art and science based medicine. Acupuncture is so ancient in theory and principles, that it is very hard to meld the energetic language and rationalization of it into a Western medicine context.

Based on this, there is no standardized acupuncture protocol for fibromyalgia patients. Also, in TCM your acupuncture treatment will depend on your "constitution". This concept of our own individual "constitution" is based on inherited/genetic factors and the unique physical and mental health state we are in at the time of treatment. The keynote here is that every patient is different. Hence, your Naturopathic Doctor may not pick the same acupuncture points for you as the points that I get needled in my own biweekly acupuncture treatment sessions.

From my own fibromyalgia battle to treating all sorts of fibromyalgia patients over the years in my private practice, I have compiled a list of key acupuncture points. These create the foundation of a solid fibromyalgia syndrome TCM protocol. The point selections discussed are based on available research, TCM teachings and mainly my own clinical experience. I encourage you to share these points with your health care provider and perhaps, they will incorporate them into your treatment plan. Also, please note that I have only provided general locations for each point below.

Acupuncture Point: Yingtang
Location: Midpoint at the glabella/between the eyebrows.
Indication: This point has been used to decrease frontal head pain and to treat insomnia and anxiety[413].

Acupuncture Point: Lung 5 (Lu5, Chize)

Location: By the cubital crease above the inner forearm. At the radial side of the biceps brachii tendon.

Indication: Some uses for this point include: Pain in the upper arm and shoulder, spasm-like pain in the elbow and arm, abdominal distension, pain in the rib area, cough, and asthma[414].

Acupuncture Point: Liver 3 (Lv3, Taichong)

Location: On top of the foot, in-between the first and second toes.

Indication: Headache, insomnia, depression, spasmodic pain, soreness in the ankle joint, abdominal pain, dizziness, and vertigo[415].

Acupuncture Point: Large Intestine 4 (Li4, Hegu)

Location: Between the thumb and the index finger.

Indication: Neck pain, redness and swelling of the eye, headache, general body and muscle pain, runny nose, and sore throat[416].

Note: This point should not be needled during pregnancy.

Acupuncture Point: Pericardium 6 (Pc6, Neiguan)

Location: On the inner forearm between the flexor radialis and palmaris longus muscles.

Indication: Stomach ache and nausea, mental health disorders, insomnia, irritable mood, pain in abdomen region, chest pain, cancer pain, hiccups and vomiting etc[417].

Acupuncture Point: San Jiao 5 (SJ5, Waiguan)

Location: On the outer forearm, in between the ulna and radius.

Indication: Headache, fever, pain in the eye, ringing in the ears, spasm and pain in the arms and shoulders, pain in the upper part of the abdomen, nerve damage[418].

Acupuncture Point: Large Intestine 15 (Li15, Jianyu)

Location: At the shoulder on the deltoid muscle.

Indication: Chronic shoulder pain, problems moving the shoulders, paralysis of the arms, swelling of glands[419].

Acupuncture Point: Gallbladder 34 (Gb34, Yanglingquan)
Location: Near the head of the fibula in the lower leg.
Indication: Pain in the shoulder, weakness in the legs, numbness and pain anywhere between the hips to the toes, knee osteo-arthritis[420].

Acupuncture Point: Stomach 24 (St24, Huaroumen)
Location: On the upper abdomen.
Indication: Psychological distress such as mania, psychosis, epigastric pain, anxiety and depression[421].

Acupuncture Point: Gallbladder 21 (Gb21, Jianjing)
Location: On the shoulder.
Indication: Headaches, neck stiffness, back pain, tense shoulders, dizziness etc[422].

Acupuncture Point: Stomach 36 (St36, Zusanli)
Location: On the front of the leg, at the outer border of the shin bone.
Indication: Abdominal pain and gastrointestinal problems, body pain, stress, nausea and fatigue[423].

Acupuncture Point: Conception Vessel 4 (CV4, Guan Yuan)
Location: On the lower abdomen.
Indication: impotence, infertility, hormonal imbalance, irregular periods, diarrhea, gas and bloating etc[424].

Acupuncture Point: Urinary Bladder 20 (UB20, Pishu)
Location: On the back.
Indication: Swelling from injury or inflammation, abdominal bloating, bloody stools, diarrhea, feeling fatigued, tired and heavy etc[425].

Myofascial Trigger Point Release on the upper back and shoulders.
Location: Wherever there is muscle pain and tenderness. Most commonly performed on the neck, upper back and shoulders.

This includes the trapezius and rhomboid muscles.

Indication: Myofascial pain therapy is different from constitutional acupuncture. There are over 350 classic acupuncture points (some of which we have listed above in our protocol). For myofascial pain therapy, we do not needle any of these points specifically. Instead, during myofascial trigger point release, your acupuncturist will find tender spots in the muscles at random and needle them through the skin[426]. Sometimes, this can cause the muscle to jump or twitch and then relax in response to the dry needling.

Think of your muscles as a mass, made up of lots of long, thick and stringy fibers or tubes. Imagine a tight, sore muscle with "knots" in it, where the fibers are tangled and tightly wound. Now imagine a needle entering one of these "knots" and causing a release, allowing the fibers to once again line up smoothly, in a detangled and relaxed order. This is kind of how active myofascial trigger point release works.

Releasing these trigger points in the muscle can help ease pain[427]. Myofascial trigger point release on the upper back is something I always add to my patients' acupuncture treatments, as I find many fibromyalgia sufferers carry tension and pain here.

CASE STUDIES: A FEW REAL-LIFE EXAMPLES.

The following are some real life fibromyalgia patient cases. The names and particular details have been changed for confidentiality reasons. I decided to add these cases into the book (with patient permission) to demonstrate that there is hope for us all. Each fibromyalgia patient is unique, but there is a buffet of different treatment options available.

Case 1
DL, a 31 year old woman diagnosed with fibromyalgia. This patient presented with positive tender points, fatigue, body aches, low mood and obesity.
Relevant Blood Work: Thyroid Stimulating Hormone Levels are low. Vitamin D deficiency.
Past Health History: Irregular weight changes. Low self-esteem and past grief surrounding a break-up. Family history of obesity and diabetes. Irregular periods.
Treatment: She was prescribed thyroid hormone therapy (Levothyroxine). Supplemented with a B-complex and given vitamin D3. Dietary changes and a daily walking exercise regimen were also implemented. DL, lost weight and experienced reduced pain within 3 months of beginning treatment. She had an increase in energy within the first 2 weeks of dietary and supplement interventions.

Case 2
RH, a 45 year old woman and mother of two, presents with IBS, headaches, chronic pain and fatigue. She was diagnosed with

fibromyalgia by a Rheumatologist, 6 months after giving birth to her second child a year ago.

Relevant Blood Work: Serum B12 levels are low. ESR and other inflammatory markers are slightly elevated. All other blood work is normal.

Past Health History: Post partum depression after the recent birth of her child. A family history of cancer and autoimmune disease on her mother's side. RH drinks 4 large cups of coffee a day.

Treatment: Gradual elimination of caffeine from her diet resulted in a 70% decrease in pain and digestive discomfort. This patient also adopted a gluten-free diet and began swimming 4 times a week. She received 2 acupuncture sessions per week for fibromyalgia pain for a total of 4 months. Supplements taken included: Relora, probiotics, l-glutamine, glucosamine, chondroitin and fish oils. At her 6 month check up, RH presented with no signs of inflammation in her blood work. Her stools became regular and well formed. Her headaches are now a very rare occurrence. RH still manages her fibromyalgia pain with low-impact aqua exercises. She continues to live a gluten-free and caffeine-free lifestyle.

Case 3

FB, a 53 year old male tested positive for fibromyalgia. He was diagnosed 15 years ago. He notes feeling heavy and sore throughout his whole body. FB also admits he consumes a lot of sugar and loves to eat pasta and bread with every meal. He feels stressed by his job as an accountant and binge eats when he is anxious. Even though it aggravates his muscle pain, he lifts heavy weights 4 times a week at the gym to "clear his mind" and counteract his high carb diet.

Relevant Blood Work: Boderline low T3 thyroid hormone levels. High HA1C (pre-diabetic).

Past Health History: Daily use of over the counter pain killers for over 10 years. He lost his first born child, who drowned at the age of 5 on a family vacation, about 15 years ago.

Treatment: FB is given a high protein and green vegetable rich diet. He replaced all the additional sugar added to his diet with stevia and monkfruit sweeteners. FB is prescribed Relora and a Bcomplex with 150mg of Rhodiola in it. He also begins taking Ashwaganda and a mineral formula of magnesium, manganese and zinc to support his thyroid. Twice a week he replaces weight lifting with Qi gong or yoga classes at his local gym. He enters into CBT therapy with a psychologist to address his unresolved grief surrounding the death of his child. Within 6 months of beginning treatment his blood work normalizes and he reports less pain and stress.

Case 5
ST is a 22 year old female, college student diagnosed with fibromyalgia. She notes having trouble concentrating at school due to mental fog and physical pain and fatigue. Sometimes her upper back and neck get so stiff that she cannot read her textbooks. She reports having low mood frequently. Often the people around her will trigger her into a state of sadness. ST admits to being hypersensitive and often comparing herself to others, especially female celebrities and models on social media. ST is sedentary but within a healthy weight range for her height and age. She suffers from insomnia and will stay up all night having negative thoughts and fears over her academic future. She often will also stay up late to party and binge-drink with her college roommates.
Relevant Blood Work: Low serum B12 and elevated liver enzymes (ALT).
Past Health History: Patient has followed a vegan diet since she was 15 years of age. No other relevant health history noted.
Treatment: ST is discouraged from drinking alcohol, as it is affecting her liver negatively. She is enrolled into a weekly meditation class and follows a meditation-yoga video at home, after school each day. She is given 50mg of 5HTP twice a day which she reports helps in elevating her mood and lowering her pain. A set of broad spectrum probiotics are also prescribed to

her. In our clinic, ST is first given a series of B12 injections to address the deficiency. After, she remains vegan but takes sublingual B12 supplements regularly. She is also given malic acid and magnesium for her muscle pain, which works well for her. ST notes after one semester being able to concentrate better in school. She also ranks lower on depression scale measurements now; and says she feels happier mentally. ST still periodically takes melatonin when she experiences bouts of insomnia brought on by academic stress.

F*CK FIBROMYALGIA

I have taken up enough of your time, so I will stay brief in concluding this book.

Firstly, I want to thank and congratulate you for taking the time to read this. Taking ownership and control over our health is no easy feat. I really hope over the next month you will be able fine tune the information I have presented here, and fit it into your lifestyle based on your individual symptom picture. It is time to begin implementing the changes and putting in the effort to heal your body. Please work with your healthcare professional. Please refer back to this text and your notes as frequently as possible. Please stay motivated. Let's go! I believe in you! The time has come to finally find reprieve from this crippling disease and shout F*CK fibromyalgia!

Yours in health,

Earth Doctor

---

[1] Vinent A, Lahr BD, Wolfe F, Clauw DJ, Whipple MO, Oh TH, Barton DL, St. Sauver J. (2013). Prevalence of fibromyalgia: a population-based study in Olmsted County, Minnesota, utilizing the Rochester Epidemiology Project. *Arthritis Care Res 65,*786–792

[2] Clauw D, Arnold L, McCarberg B. (2011). The Science of Fibromyalgia. *Mayo Clin. Proc.* 86, 907 – 911.

[3] Arnold LM, Crofford LJ, Mease PJ, Burgess SM, Palmer SC, Abetz L, Martin SA. (2008). Patient Perspectives on The Impact of Fibromyalgia. *Patient Educ Couns. 73(1):114-20.*

[4] Goldenberg DL, Schaefer CR, Ryan K, Chandran A, Slateva G. What is The True Cost of Fibromyalgia to Our Society: Results From a Cross-sectional Survey in the United States. Paper presented at: *American College of Rheumatology.* Philadelphia, PA: October 18, 2009.

[5] Petzke F, Clauw DJ, Ambrose K, Khine A, Gracely RH. (2003). Increased pain sensitivity in fibromyalgia: effects of stimulus type and mode of presentation. *Pain 105(3),* 403–413.

[6] Gracely RH, Petzke F, Wolf JM, Clauw DJ. (2002). Functional magnetic resonance imaging evidence of augmented pain processing in fibromyalgia. *Arthritis and Rheumatology. 46*(5). 1333–1343.

[7] Berger M, Gray JA, Roth BL (2009). "The expanded biology of serotonin". *Annual Review of Medicine 60, 355–366.*

[8] Hasler, W.L. (2009). Serotonin and the GI tract. *Current Gastroenerology Reports* 11(5), 383-391

[9] Russel, IJ. (1999). Neurochemical pathogenesis of fibromyalgia syndrome. *Journal of Musculoskeletal Pain 7, 183-191.*

[10] Wolfe F, Russell IJ, Vipraio G, Ross K, Anderson J. (1997). Serotonin levels, pain threshold, and fibromyalgia symptoms in the general population. *Journal of Rheumatology 24*(3), 555–559.

[11] Yunus MB, Dailey JW, Aldag JC, Masi AT, Jobe PC. (1992). Plasma tryptophan and other amino acids in primary fibromyalgia: a controlled study. *Journal of Rheumatology 19*(1), 90–94.

[12] Russel, IJ., Vaeroy, H., Javors, M., et al. (1992). Cerebrospinal fluid biogenic amine metabolites in fibromyalgia/fibrositis syndrome and rheumatoid arthritis. *Arthritis Rheumatology 35*, 550-556.

[13] O'Malley, PG., Balden, E., Tomkins, G. et al. (2000). Treatment of fibromyalgia with antidepressants a meta-analysis. *Journal of General Internal Medicine 15, 659-666.*

[14] Bennet, RM. (2002). Antidepressants do not have better results than placebo in the treatment of fibromyalgia in Brazil. *Current Rheumotology Reports 4*, 282-285.

[15] Arnold LM, Hess EV, Hudson JI, Welge JA, Berno SE, Keck PE Jr. (2002) A randomized, placebo-controlled, double-blind, flexible-dose study of fluoxetine in the treatment of women with fibromyalgia. *American Journal of Medicine 112*(3), 191–197.

[16] Lowe, JC. (2002). The metabolic treatment of fibromyalgia. Boulder, CO: McDowell Publishing.

[17] Lowe, JC. and Honeyman-Lowe G. (2000). Thyroid disease and fibromyalgia syndrome. *Lyon Mediterranee Medical: Medecine du Sud-Est 36, 15-17.*

[18] Honeyman, GS. (1997). Metabolic therapy for hypothyroid and euthyroid fibromyalgia: two case reports. *Clinical Bulletin of Myofascial Therapy 2*, 19-49.

[19] Lowe, JC. (1997). Results of an open trial of T3 therapy with 77 euthyroid female fibromyalgia patients. *Clinical Bulletin of Myofascial Therapy 2*, 35-37.

[20] Lowe, JC., Reichman, AJ., and Yellin, J. (1998). A case-control study of metabolic therapy for fibromyalgia: Long-term follow-up comparison of treated and untreated patients. *Clinical Bulletin of Myofascial Therapy 3*, 65-79.

[21] Lowe, JC. (1997). Results of an open trial of T3 therapy with 77 euthyroid female fibromyalgia patients. *Clinical Bulletin of Myofascial Therapy 2*, 35-37.

[22] Vaeroy, H., Helle, R., Forre, O. et al. (1988). Elevated CSF levels of substance P and high incidence of Raynaud phenomenon in patients with fibromyalgia: new features for diagnosis. *Pain 32*, 21-26.

[23] Mendelson, SC. And Quinn, JP. (1995). Characterization of potential regulatory elements within the rat preprotachykinin-A promoter. *Neuroscience Letters 184*, 125-128.

[24] Too, HP., Marriott, DR. and Wilkin, GP. (1994). Preportachykinin-A and substance preceptor (NK1) gene expression in rat astrocytes in vitro. *Neuroscience Letters 182*, 185-187.

[25] Hammond, DL. (1986). Control systems for nociceptive afferent processing; the descending inhibitory pathways. In Yaksh TL, ed. Spinal affarant processing. New York: Plenum Press, 1986: 363-390.

[26] Pertovaara, A. (2013). The noradrenergic pain regulation system: a potential target for pain therapy. *European Journal of Pharmacology 716*(3), 2-7.

[27] Gordon, JT., Kaminski, DM., Rozanov, CB., et al. (1999). Evidence that 335-triiodothyronine is concentrated in and delivered from the locus coeruleus to its noradrenergic targets via anterograde axonal transport. *Neuroscience 6*, 943-954.

[28] Riedel, W. and Neeck, G. (2001). Nociception, pain and antinociception: current concepts. *Zeitschrift fur Rheumatologie* 60, 404-415.

[29] Dworkin, RH., Hetzel, RD., and Banks, SM. (199). Toward a model of the pathogenesis of chronic pain. *Seminars in Clinical Neuropsychiatry 4*(3), 176–185.

[30] Smith SB, Maixner DW, Fillingim RB et al. (2012). Large candidate gene association study reveals genetic risk factors and therapeutic targets for fibromyalgia. *Arthritis and Rheumatolgy 64*(2), 584–593.

[31] Harris RE, Clauw DJ, Scott DJ, Mclean SA, Gracely RH, Zubieta J-K. (2007). Decreased central μ-opioid receptor availability in fibromyalgia. *Journal of Neuroscience* 27(37), 10000–10006.

[32] Katom K., Sullivan, PF., Evengård, B. and Pedersen, NL. (2006). Importance of genetic influences on chronic widespread pain. *Arthritis and Rheumatology 54*(5), 1682–1686.

[33] Manuel, ML. (2007). Biology and therapy of fibromyalgia. Stress, the stress response system, and fibromyalgia. *Arthritis Research and Therapy 9*(4), 216–216.

[34] Zubieta, JK., Heitzeg, MM., Smith, YR. et al. (2003) *COMT* val158met genotype affects mu-opioid neurotransmitter responses to a pain stressor. *Science 299*(5610), 1240–1243.

[35] Desmeules, J., Piguet, V., Besson, M. et al. (2012). Psychological distress in fibromyalgia patients: a role for catechol- *O* -methyl-transferase Val158met polymorphism. *Health Psychology 31*(2), 242–249.

[36] Aguglia, A., Salvi, V., Maina, G., Rossetto, I. and Aguglia, E. (2011). Fibromyalgia syndrome and depressive symptoms: comorbidity and clinical correlates. *Journal of Affective Disorders.128*(3), 262–266.

[37] Stisi, S., Venditti, C. and Sarracco, I. (2008). Distress influence in fibromyalgia. *Reumatismo 60*(4), 274–281.

[38] Malin, Katrina and Littlejohn, Geoffrey. (2012). Personality and fibromyalgia syndrome. *The Open Rheumatology Journal 6*, 273-285.

[39] Soderberg, S., Lundman, B. and Norberg, A. (1997). Living with fibromyalgia: sense of coherence, perception of well-being, and stress in daily life. *Research in Nursing and Health 20*, 495–503.

[40] Johannsson, V. (1993). Does a Fibromyalgia Personality Exist? *Journal of Musculoskeletal Pain 1*, 245–252.

[41] Magnusson, AE., Nias, DK. and White, PD. (1996). Is perfectionism associated with fatigue? *Journal of Psychosomatic Research 41*(4), 377-383.

[42] Herken, H., Gursoy, S., Yetkin, OE., Virit, O. and Esgi, K. (2001). Personality characteristics and depression level of the female patients with fibromyalgia syndrome. *Internal Medicine Journal 8*, 41–44.

[43] Kendall, SA., Elert, J., Ekselius, L. and Gerdle, B. (2002).Are perceived muscle tension, electromyographic hyperactivity and personality traits correlated in the fibromyalgia syndrome? *Journal of Rehabilitation Medicine 34*(2), 73-79.

[44] Kamping, S., Bomba, IC., Kanske, P., Diesch, E. and Flor, H. (2013). Deficient modulation of pain by a positive emotional context in fibromyalgia patients. *Pain 154*(9), 1846–1855.

[45] Amir, M., Neuman, L., Bor, O., Shir, Y., Rubinow, A. and Buskila, D. (2000). Coping styles, Anger, Social Support, and Suicide Risk of Women with Fibromyalgia. *Journal of Musculoskeletal Pain* 8, 7-20.

[46] Conrad, R., Schilling. G., Bausch, C., Nadstawek, J., Wartenberg, HC., Wegener, I., Geiser, F., Imbierowicz, K. and Liedtke, R. (2007). Temperament and character personality profiles and personality disorders in chronic pain patients. *Pain 133*, 197-209.

[47] Hannibal, KE. And Bishop, MD. (2014). Chronic stress, cortisol dysfunction, and pain: a psychoneuroendocrine rationale for stress management in pain rehabilitation. *Physical Therapy 12*, 1816-1825.

[48] Nemeroff, CB. and Vale, WW. (2005). The neurobiology of depression: inroads to treatment and new drug discovery. *The Journal of Clinical Psychiatry 7*, 5-13.

[49] Binder, EB. And Holsboer, F. (2012). Low cortisol and risk and resilience to stress-related psychiatric disorders. *Biological Psychiatry* 71(4), 282-283.

[50] Camilla A.M., Glad, J., C. Andersson-Assarsson, Berglund, P., Ragnhildur B., Ragnarsson, O. and Gudmundur, J. (2017). Reduced DNA methylation and psychopathology following endogenous hypercortisolism – a genome-wide study. *Scientific Reports, 7*, 444-445.

[51] Leproult, R., Copinshchi, G., Buxton, O. and Van Cauter, E. (1997). American Sleep Disorders Association and Sleep Research Society Sleep Loss Sleep Loss Results in an Elevation of Cortisol Levels the Next Evening. *Sleep 20*(10), 865-870.

[52] Pecoraro, N., Reyes, F., Gomez, F., Bhargava, A. and Dallman, MF. (2004). Chronic stress promotes palatable feeding, which reduces signs of stress: feedforward and feedback effects of chronic stress. *Endocrinology* 145(8), 3754-3762.

[53] Rutters, F., Nieuwenhuizen, AG., Lemmens, SG., Born, JM. and Westerterp-Plantenga, MS. (2009). Acute stress-related changes in eating in the absence of hunger. *Obesity 17*(1), 72-77.

[54] Office of Disease Prevention and Health Promotion, 2015 Dietary Guidelines Advisory Committee. Scientific Report of the 2015 Dietary Guidelines Advisory Committee. Washington (DC): Office of Disease Prevention and Health Promotion; 2015.

[55] Kumamoto, C. (2011). Inflammation and gastrointestinal Candida colonization. *Current Opinions in Microbiology 14*(4), 386-391.

[56] Marijnissen, RJ., Koenders, MI., van de Veerdonk, FL., Dulos, J., Netea, MG., Boots, AM., Joosten, LA. and van den Berg, WB. (2012). Exposure to Candida albicans polarizes a T-cell driven arthritis model towards TH17 responses, resulting in more destructive arthritis. *PloS ONE 7*(6), e38889.

[57] Irfan, S., Rani, A., Naila, R., Muhammad, A. and Sayed, KN. (2017). Comparative evaluation of heavy metals in patients with rheumatoid arthritis and healthy control in Pakistani population. *Iranian Journal of Public Health 46*(5), 626-633.

[58] Felsby, S. Nielsen, J., Arendt-Nielsen, L. and Jensen, TS. (1996). NMDA receptor blockade in chronic neuropathic pain: a comparison of ketamine and magnesium chloride. *Pain 64*(2), 283-291.

[59] Clauw, D. And Sluka, K. (2016). Neurobiology of fibromyalgia and chronic widespread pain. *Neuroscience 338*, 114-129.

[60] Holton, KF., Taren, DL. Thomson, CA., Bennet, RM. And Jones, KD. (2012). The effect of dietary glutamate on fibromyalgia and irritable bowel symptoms. *Clinical and Experimental Rheumatology 6*, 10-17.

[61] Van den Eaden, SK., Koepsell, TD., Longstreth, WT., van Belle, G., Daling, JR. And McKnight, B. (1994). Aspartame ingestion and headaches: a randomized crossover trial. *Neurology 44*(10), 1787-1793.

[62] Boston, MA: Harvard School of Public Health Nutrition Source; 2011. [Accessed 10

January 2017]. Healty Eating Plate and Healthy Eating Pyramid. Available from: https://www.hsph.harvard.edu/nutritionsource/healthy-eating-plate/

[63] Melnik, B. (2009). Milk–the promoter of chronic Western diseases. *Medical Hypotheses 72*, 631–639.

[64] Segura-jimenez, V., Alvarez-gallardo, IC., Estevez-lopez, F. et al. (2015). Differences in Sedentary Time and Physical Activity Between Female Patients with Fibromyalgia and Healthy Controls: The al-Andalus Project. *Arthritis and Rheumatology 67*(11), 3047-3057.

[65] Norregaard, J., Lykkegaard, JJ., Mehlsen, J. et al. (1996). Exercise Training in Treatment of Fibromyalgia. *Journal of Musculoskeletal Pain 5*, 71-79.

[66] Mengshoel, AM. and Forre, O. (1993). Physical Fitness Training in Patients with Fibromyalgia. *Journal of Musculoskeletal Pain 1*, 267-272.

[67] Meiworm, L., Jakob, E., Walker, UA., Peter, HH. and Keul, J. (2000). Patients with Fibromyalgia Benefit from Aerobic Endurance Exercise. *Clinical Rheumatology 19*(4), 253-257.

[68] Fernandes, G., Jennings, F., Nery Cabral, MV., Buosi Pirozzi, AL. and Natour, J. (2016). Swimming Improves Pain and Functional Capacity of Patients with Fibromyalgia: A Randomized Controlled Trial. *Archives of Physical Medicine and Rehabilitation 97*(8), 1269-1275.

[69] Ericsson, A., Palstam, A., Larsson, A. et al. (2016). Resistance Exercise Improves Physical Fatigue in Women with Fibromyalgia: A Randomized Controlled Trial. *Arthritis Research and Therapy 18*, 176.

[70] Wolfe, F., Clauw, DJ., Fitzcharles, M., Goldenberg, R., Katz, R., Mease, P., Russel, A., Russel, J., Winfield, J. and Yunus, M. (2010). The American College of Rheumatology Preliminary Diagnostic Criteria for Fibromyalgia and Measurement of Symptom Severity. *Arthritis Care and Research 62*(5), 600-610.

[71] Sarma PR. Red Cell Indices. In: Walker HK, Hall WD, Hurst JW, editors. Clinical Methods: The History, Physical, and Laboratory Examinations. 3rd edition. Boston: Butterworths; 1990. Chapter 152. Available from: https://www.ncbi.nlm.nih.gov/books/NBK260/

[72] Haliloglu, S., Ekinci, B., Uzkeser, H., Sevimli, H., Carlioglu, A. and Macit, PM. (2017). Fibromyalgia in Patients with Thyroid Autoimmunity Prevalence and Relationship with Disease Activity. *Clinical Rheumatology 36*(7), 1617-1621.

[73] Armughan, A., Rehman, M. and Saeed, M. (2017). Rheumatoid Arthritis Masquerading as Fibromyalgia. *Journal of the College of Physicians and Surgeons Pakistan 27*, 134-136.

[74] Xiao, Y., Haynes, WL., Michalek, JE. and Russell, IJ. (2013). Elevated Serum High-Sensitivity C-reactive Protein Levels in Fibromyalgia Syndrome Patients Correlate with Body Mass Index, Interleukin-6, Interleukin-8, Erythrocyte Sedimentation Rate. *Rheumatology International 33*(5), 1259-1264.

[75] Akkus, S., Senol, A., Ayyacioglu, NB., Tunc, E., Eren, I. and Isler, M. (2004). Is Female Predominance in Irritable Bowel Syndrome Related to Fibromyalgia. *Rheumatology International 24*(2), 106-109.

[76] Whitehead, WE., Palsson, O. and Jones, KR. (2002). Systematic Review of the Comorbidity of Irritable Bowel Syndrome with Other Disorders: What are the causes and implications? *Gastroenterology 122*(4), 1140-1156.

[77] Jadallah, KA. Nimri, LF. and Ghanem, RA. (2017). Protozoan Parasites in Irritable Bowel Syndrome: A Case-Control Study. *World Journal of Gastrointestinal Pharmacology and Therapeutics 8*(4), 201-207.

[78] Nisihara, R., Marques, AP., Mei, A. and Skare, T. (2016). Celiac disease and fibromyalgia: Is there an association? *Revista Española de Enfermedades Digestivas 108*(2), 107-108.

[79] Isasi, C., Colmenero, I., Casco, F., Tejerina, E., Fernandez, N., Serrano-Vela, J., Castro, M. and Villa, L. (2014). Fibromyalgia and non-celiac gluten sensitivity: a description with remission of fibromyalgia. *Rheumatology International 34*(11). 1607-1612.

[80] Benson, B. C., Mulder, C. J., & Laczek, J. T. (2013). Anti-Gliadin Antibodies Identify Celiac Patients Overlooked by Tissue Transglutaminase Antibodies. *Hawai'i Journal of Medicine & Public Health, 72*(9), 14–17.

[81] Levine, TD. and Saperstein, DS. (2015). Routine use of punch biopsy to diagnose small fiber neuropathy in fibromyalgia patients. *Clinical Rheumatology 34*(3), 413-417.

[82] Keyes, RD. (1990). Nerve Conduction Studies and Electromyography. *Canadian Family Physician 36*, 317-320.

[83] Maquet, D., Croisier, JL., Dupont, C., Moutschen, M., Ansseau, M., Zeevaert, B. And Crielaard, JM. (2010). Fibromyalgia and Related Conditions: Electromyogram profile during isometric muscle contraction. *Joint Bone Spine 77*(3), 264-267.

[84] Oaklander, AL., Herzog, ZD., Downs, HM. and Klein, MM. (2013). Objective evidence that small-fiber polyneuropathy underlies some illnesses currently labelled as fibromyalgia. *Pain 154*(11), 2310-2316.

[85] Dzugan, SA. and Dzugan KS.(2015). Is migraine a consequence of a loss of neurohormonal and metabolic integrity? A new hypothesis. *Neuro Enfrocrinology Letters 36*(5), 421-429.

[86] Eiching, PS. and Sahni, J. (2005). Menopause related sleep disorders. *Journal of Clinical Sleep Medicine 15*(3), 291-300.

[87] Schertzinger, M., Wesson-Sides, K., Parkitny, L. and Younger, J. (2018). *Journal of Pain 19*(4), 410-417.

[88] Gur, A., Cevik, R., Sarac, AJ., Colpan, L. and Em, S. (2004). Hypothalamic-pituitary-gonadal axis and cortisol in young women with primary fibromyalgia: the potential roles of depression, fatigue, and sleep disturbance in the occurrence of hypocortisolism. *Annals of the Rheumatic Diseases 63*(11), 1504-1506.

[89] Gur, A., Cevik, R., Nas, K., Colpan, L. and Sarac, S. (2004). Cortisol and hypothalamic-pituitary-gonadal axis hormones in follicular-phase women with fibromyalgia and chronic fatigue syndrome and effect of depressive symptoms on these hormones. *Arthritis Research Therapy 6*(3), 232-238.

[90] Cadegiani, F. A., & Kater, C. E. (2016). Adrenal fatigue does not exist: a systematic review. *BMC Endocrine Disorders, 16*(1), 48.

[91] Moshe, T., Tatyana, S., Mirit, VA., Yoram, R., Michael, K., Beno, F. (2003). Fibromyalgia in diabetes mellitus. *Rheumatology International 23*(4). 171-173.

[92] May, KP., West, SG., Baker, MR. and Everett, DW. (1993). Sleep apnea in male patients with the fibromyalgia syndrome. *American Journal of Medicine 94*(5), 505-508.

[93] Martinez, D. And Cassol CM. (2008). Fibromyalgia and sleep-disordered breathing: the missing link. *Arthritis Research and Therapy 10*, 408.

[94] Gota CE, Jhala N, Kaouk S, Kinanah Y, Wilke W. (2018). Sleep Apnea and Fibromyalgia: Data from the Cleveland Clinic Fibromyalgia Registry. *Arthritis Rheumatology 70* (10). https://acrabstracts.org/abstract/sleep-apnea-and-fibromyalgia-data-from-the-cleveland-clinic-fibromyalgia-registry/. Accessed October 10, 2018.

[95] Ortancil, O., Sanli, A., Eryuksel, R., Basaran, A. and Ankarali, H. (2010). Association between serum ferritin level and fibromyalgia syndrome. *European Journal of Clinical Nutrition 64*(3), 308-312.

[96] Gröber, U., Kisters, K., & Schmidt, J. (2013). Neuroenhancement with Vitamin B12—Underestimated Neurological Significance. *Nutrients, 5*(12), 5031–5045.

[97] Gupta, L., Gupta, RK., Gupta, PK. , Malhotra, HS., Saha, I. and Garg, RK. (2016). Assessment of brain cognitive functions in patients with vitamin B12 deficiency using resting state functional MRI: A longitudinal study. *Magnetic Resonance Imaging 34*(2), 191-196.

[98] Oberlin, B. S., Tangney, C. C., Gustashaw, K. A. R., & Rasmussen, H. E. (2013). Vitamin B12 Deficiency in Relation to Functional Disabilities. *Nutrients, 5*(11), 4462–4475.

[99] Regland, B., Forsmark, S., Halaouate, L., Matousek, M., Peilot, B., Zachrisson, O. and Gottfries, CG. (2015). Response to vitamin B12 and folic acid in myalgic encephalomyelitis and fibromyalgia. *PLoS One 10*(4), e0124648.

[100] Yang, G.-T., Zhao, H.-Y., Kong, Y., Sun, N.-N., & Dong, A.-Q. (2018). Correlation between serum vitamin B12 level and peripheral neuropathy in atrophic gastritis. *World Journal of Gastroenterology, 24*(12), 1343–1352.

[101] Bikle, D. And Bouillon, R. (2018). Vitamin D and muscle. *Bone Reports 8*, 163-167.

[102] Shipton, E. E., & Shipton, E. A. (2015). Vitamin D Deficiency and Pain: Clinical Evidence of Low Levels of Vitamin D and Supplementation in Chronic Pain States. *Pain and Therapy, 4*(1), 67–87.

[103] Stewart, AE., Roecklein, KA., Tanner, S. And Kimlin, MG. (2014). *Medical Hypotheses 83*(5), 517-525.

[104] Eleni, R., Stauros, M. and Kalliopi, K. (2016). Vitamin D in Fibromyalgia: A causative or confounding biological interplay? *Nutrients 8*(6), 343.

[105] Makrani, AH., Afshari, M., Ghajar, M., Forooghi, Z. and Moosazadeh, M. (2017). Vitamin D and fibromyalgia: a meta-analysis. *Korean Journal of Pain 30*(4), 250-257.

[106] Dogru, A., Balkarli, A., Cobankara, V., Tunc, S. E., and Sahin, M. (2017). Effects of Vitamin D Therapy on Quality of Life in Patients with Fibromyalgia. *The Eurasian Journal of Medicine, 49*(2), 113–117.

[107] De Carvalho, JF., Da Rocha, AF., Da Mota, LMA., Aires, RB. and De Araujo, RP. (2018). Vitamin D supplementation seems to improve fibromyalgia symptoms: Preliminary Results. *The Israel Medical Association Journal 20*(6), 379-381.

[108] Forte ML, Butler M, Andrade KE, et al. Treatments for Fibromyalgia in Adult Subgroups [Internet]. Rockville (MD): Agency for Healthcare Research and Quality (US); 2015 Jan. (Comparative Effectiveness Reviews, No. 148.) Table 1, FDA-approved drugs for the treatment of fibromyalgia. Available from: https://www.ncbi.nlm.nih.gov/books/NBK274463/table/introduction.t1

[109] Dayan, C., & Panicker, V. (2018). Management of hypothyroidism with combination thyroxine (T4) and triiodothyronine (T3) hormone replacement in clinical practice: a review of suggested guidance. *Thyroid research, 11*, 1.

[110] Chung H. R. (2014). Iodine and thyroid function. *Annals of pediatric endocrinology & metabolism, 19*(1), 8-12.

[111] Khaliq, W., Andreis, D. T., Kleyman, A., Gräler, M., & Singer, M. (2015). Reductions in tyrosine levels are associated with thyroid hormone and catecholamine disturbances in sepsis. *Intensive Care Medicine Experimental, 3*(Suppl 1), A686.

[112] Jongkees, BJ., Hommel, B., Kuhn, S. And Colzato, LS. (2015). Effect of tyrosine supplementation on clinical and healthy populations under stress or cognitive demands. A review. *Journal of Psychiatric Research 70*, 50-57.

[113] Dailly, E., Chenu, F., Renard, C. And Bourin, M. (2004). Dopamine, depression and antidepressants. *Fundamentals and Clinical Pharmacology 18*(6), 601-607.

[114] Van de Rest, O., Bloemendaal, M., De Heus, R. And Aarts, E. (2017). Dose-Dependent Effects of Oral Tyrosine Administration on Plasma Tyrosine Levels and Cognition in Aging. *Nutrients 9*(12), 1-14.

[115] Young S. N. (2007). L-tyrosine to alleviate the effects of stress?. *Journal of psychiatry & neuroscience 32*(3), 224.

[116] Laurberg, P. (1984). Forskolin Stimulation of Thyroid Secretion of T4 and T3. *FEEBS Letters 170*(2), 273-276.

[117] Ammon, H.P., and Muller, A.B., "Forskolin: From an Ayurvedic Remedy to a Modern Agent," Planta Med Dec.6 (1985) : 473-7.

[118] Godard MP, Johnson BA, Richmond SR. Body composition and hormonal adaptations associated with forskolin consumption in overweight and obese men. Obes Res. 2005;13:1335–1343.

[119] Singh, N., Bhalla, M., de Jager, P., & Gilca, M. (2011). An overview on ashwagandha: a Rasayana (rejuvenator) of Ayurveda. *African journal of traditional, complementary, and alternative medicines : AJTCAM, 8*(5 Suppl), 208-13.

[120] Sharma, AK., Basu, I. and Singh, S. (2018). Efficacy and Safety of Ashwagandha Root Extract in Subclinical Hypothyroid Patients: A Double-Blind, Randomized Placebo-Controlled Trial. *Journal of Alternative and Complementary Medicine 24*(3), 243-248.

[121] Leung, H. W., Foo, G., Banumurthy, G., Chai, X., Ghosh, S., Mitra-Ganguli, T., & VanDongen, A. (2017). The effect of Bacopa monnieri on gene expression levels in SH-SY5Y human neuroblastoma cells. *PloS one, 12*(8), e0182984.

[122] Kar A, Panda S, Bharti S. Relative efficacy of three medicinal plant extracts in the alteration of thyroid hormone concentrations in male mice. J Ethnopharmacol. 2002 Jul;81(2):281-5.

[123] Shahid, M., Subhan, F., Ahmad, N., & Ullah, I. (2017). A bacosides containing Bacopa monnieri extract alleviates allodynia and hyperalgesia in the chronic constriction injury model of neuropathic pain in rats. *BMC complementary and alternative medicine, 17*(1), 293.

[124] Neupane, N., Kaur, M. and Pranav, P. (2017). Treatment of Hashimoto's thyroiditis with herbal medication. *International Journal of Green Pharmacy 11*(3), 343-347.

[125] Culpeper. 1995. *Culpeper's Complete Herbal.* Great Britain: Wordsworth Editions Ltd.

[126] Chevallier A. 2001. *Encyclopedia of Medicinal Plants.* St Leonards NSW: Dorling Kindersley.

[127] Kunnumakkara, Ajaikumar B et al. "Googling the Guggul (Commiphora and Boswellia) for Prevention of Chronic Diseases" *Frontiers in pharmacology* vol. 9 686. 6 Aug. 2018.

[128] Deng, R., Yang, D., Radke, A., Yang, J., & Yan, B. (2006). The hypolipidemic agent guggulsterone regulates the expression of human bile salt export pump: dominance of transactivation over farsenoid X receptor-mediated antagonism. *The Journal of pharmacology and experimental therapeutics, 320*(3), 1153-62.

[129] Tripathi YB, Malhotra OP, Tripathi SN. (1984). Thyroid stimulating action of Z-guggulsterone obtained from Commiphora mukul. *Planta Med 50* (34), 78-80.

[130] Panda S, Kar A. (1999). Gugulu (Commiphora mukul) induces triiodothyronine production: Possible involvement of lipid peroxidation. *Life Sci 65*, 137-141.

[131] Stansbury J, Saunders P, Winton D. (2012). Promoting health thyroid function with iodine,

bladderwrack, guggal and Iris. *Journal of Restorative Medicine 1*, 83-90.

[132] Negro R. (2008). Selenium and thyroid autoimmunity. *Biologics : targets & therapy*, 2(2), 265-73.

[133] Bianco, A. C., & Kim, B. W. (2006). Deiodinases: implications of the local control of thyroid hormone action. *The Journal of clinical investigation*, 116(10), 2571-9.

[134] Chanoine JP. Selenium and thyroid function in infants, children and adolescents. Biofactors. 2003;19(3-4):137-43. Review.

[135] Allen, DK., Hassel, CA. and Lei, KY. (1982). Function of pituitary-thyroid axis in copper deficient rats. *The Journal of Nutrition 112*(11), 2043-2046.

[136] Jain, RB. (2014). Thyroid function and serum copper, selenium, and zinc in general US. population. *Biological Trace Element Research 159*(1-3), 87-98.

[137] Mahmoodianfard, S., Vafa, M., Golgiri, F., Khoshniat, M., Gohari, M., Solati, Z. and Djalali, M. (2015). Effects of Zinc and Selenium Supplementation on Thyroid Function in Overweight and Obese Hypothyroid Female Patients: A randomized double-blind controlled trial. *Journal of the American College of Nutrition 34*(5), 391-399.

[138] Betsy, A., Binitha, M., & Sarita, S. (2013). Zinc deficiency associated with hypothyroidism: an overlooked cause of severe alopecia. *International journal of trichology*, 5(1), 40-2.

[139] Soldin, O. P., & Aschner, M. (2007). Effects of manganese on thyroid hormone homeostasis: potential links. *Neurotoxicology*, 28(5), 951-6.

[140] Uum Van, SHM., Suave, B., Fraser, LA., Morley-Forster, P., Paul, TL. and Koren, G. (2009). Elevated content of cortisol in hair of patients with severe chronic pain: a novel biomarker for stress. *The International Journal on the Biology of Stress* 483-488.

[141] Young, E., Lopez, J., Murphy-Weinberg, V., Watson, S. And Akil, H. (2000). Hormonal Evidence for Altered Responsiveness to social stress in major depression. Neuropsychopharmacology 23(4), 411.

[142] Ranabir, S. And Reetu, K. (2011). Stress and Hormones. *Indian Journal of Endocrinology and Metabolism 15*(1), 18.

[143]Taylor, T., Robert, GD. and Williams, GH. (1983). B-Endorphin Supresses Adrenocorticotropin and Cortisol Levels in Normal Human Subjects. *The Journal of Clinical Endocrinology and Metabolism 57*(3), 592-596.

[144] Talbott, SM., Talbott, JA. and Pugh, M. (2013). Effects of Magnolia officinalis and Phellodendron amurense (Relora) on cortisol and psychological mood state in moderately stressed subjects. *Journal of the International Society of Sports Nutrition 10*(3), 37.

[145] Chen, CR. et al. (2012). Magnolol, a major bioactive constituent of the bark of Magnolia officinalis induces sleep via the benzodiazepine site of GABAA receptor in mice. *Neuropharmacology 63*, 1191-1199.

[146] Debono, M. et al. (2009). Modified-release hydrocortisone to provide circadian cortisol profiles. *The Journal of Clinical Endocrinology and Metabolism 94*(5), 1548-1554.

[147] Panossian, A. and Wikman, G. (2009). Evidence-based efficacy of adaptogens in fatigue, and molecular mechanisms related to their stress-protective activity. *Current Clinical Pharmacology 4*(3), 198-219.

[148] Panossian, A., Wikman, G. and Sarris, J. (2010). Rosenroot (Rhodiola rosea): traditional use, chemical composition, pharmacology and clinical efficacy. *Phytomedicine 17*(7), 481-493.

[149] Amsterdam, JD. And Panossian, AG. (2016). Rhodiola rosea L. as a putative botanical anti-depressant. *Phytomedicine 23*(7), 770-783.

[150] Al-Nimer, M., Mohammad, T., & Alsakeni, R. A. (2018). Serum levels of serotonin as a biomarker of newly diagnosed fibromyalgia in women: Its relation to the platelet indices. *Journal of research in medical sciences:the official journal of Isfahan University of Medical Sciences, 23*, 71.

[151] Tafet, GE., Idoyaga-Vargas, VP., Abulafia, DP., Calandria, JM., Roffman, SS., Chiovetta, A. and Shinitzky, M. (2001). Correlation between cortisol level and serotonin uptake in patients with chronic stress and depression. *Cognitive, Affective and Behavioural Neuroscience 1*(4), 388-393.

[152] Weeks, BS. (2009). Formulations of dietary supplements and herbal extracts for relaxation and anxiolytic action: Relarian. *Medical Science Monitor15*(11), 256-262.

[153] Birdsall, TC. (1998). 5-hydroxytryptophan: a clinically-effective serotonin precursor. *Alternative Medicine Review 3*(4), 271-280.

[154] Caruso I, Sarzi Puttini P, Cazzola M, Azzolini V. (1990). Double-blind study of 5-hydroxytryptophan versus placebo in the treatment of primary fibromyalgia syndrome. *J Int Med Res. 18*(3), 201-209.

[155] Juhl JH. (1998). Primary fibromyalgia syndrome and 5-hydroxy-L-tryptophan: a 90-day open study. *Altern Med Rev.3*(5), 367-375.

[156] Ribeiro, CA. (2000). L-5-hydroxytryptophan in the prophylaxis of chronic tension-type headache: a double-blind, randomized, placebo-controlled study. *Headache* 40(6), 451-456.

[157] Shaw K, Turner J, Del Mar C. (2002). Are tryptophan and 5-hydroxytryptophan effective treatments for depression? A meta-analysis. *Aust N Z J Psychiatry* 36(4), 488-491.

[158] Attele AS, Xie JT, Yuan CS. (2000). Treatment of insomnia: an alternative approach. *Altern Med Rev.* 5(3), 249-259.

[159] Cangiano C, Laviano A, Del Ben M, et al. (1998). Effects of oral 5-hydroxy-tryptophan on energy intake and macronutrient selection in non-insulin dependent diabetic patients. *Int J Obes Relat Metab Disord.* 22(7), 648-654.

[160] Inam, QU., Ikram, H., Shireen, E. and Haleem, DJ. (2016). Effects of sugar rich diet on brain serotonin, hyperphagia and anxiety in animal model of both genders. *Pakistan Journal of Pharmaceutical Sciences 29*(3), 757-763.

[161] Benloucif, S., Burgess, H. J., Klerman, E. B., Lewy, A. J., Middleton, B., Murphy, P. J., Parry, B. L. et al. (2008). Measuring melatonin in humans. *Journal of clinical sleep medicine : JCSM : official publication of the American Academy of Sleep Medicine, 4*(1), 66-9.

[162] Huang CT, Chiang RP, Chen CL, Tsai YJ. (2014). Sleep deprivation aggravates median nerve injury-induced neuropathic pain and enhances microglial activation by suppressing melatonin secretion. *SLEEP 37*(9):1513-1523.

[163] Castano, MY., Garrido, M., Rodriguez, AB. And Gomez, MA. (2018). Melatonin improves mood status and quality of life and decreases cortisol levels in Fibromyalgia. *Biological Research for Nursing.*

[164] de Zanette, SA. et al. (2014). Melatonin analgesia is associated with improvement of the descending endogenous pain-modulating system in fibromyalgia: a phase II, randomized, double-dummy, controlled trial. *BMC pharmacology & toxicology, 15*, 40.

[165] Danilov, A., & Kurganova, J. (2016). Melatonin in Chronic Pain Syndromes. *Pain and therapy, 5*(1), 1-17.

[166] Plante, D. T., Jensen, J. E., Schoerning, L., & Winkelman, J. W. (2012). Reduced γ-aminobutyric acid in occipital and anterior cingulate cortices in primary insomnia: a link to major depressive disorder?. *Neuropsychopharmacology : official publication of the American College of Neuropsy-*

chopharmacology, 37(6), 1548-57.

[167] Abdou, AM., Higashiguchi, S., Horie, K., Kim, M., Hatta, H. and Yokogoshi, H. (2006). Relaxation and immunity enhancement effects of gamma-aminobutyric acid (GABA) administration in humans. *Biofactors 26*(3), 201-208.

[168] Foerster, B. R., Petrou, M., Edden, R. A., Sundgren, P. C., Schmidt-Wilcke, T., Lowe, S. E., Harte, S. E., Clauw, D. J., ... Harris, R. E. (2012). Reduced insular γ-aminobutyric acid in fibromyalgia. *Arthritis and rheumatism, 64*(2), 579-83.

[169] Nuss P. (2015). Anxiety disorders and GABA neurotransmission: a disturbance of modulation. *Neuropsychiatric disease and treatment, 11*, 165-75.

[170] Rosso, I. M., Weiner, M. R., Crowley, D. J., Silveri, M. M., Rauch, S. L., & Jensen, J. E. (2013). Insula and anterior cingulate GABA levels in posttraumatic stress disorder: preliminary findings using magnetic resonance spectroscopy. *Depression and anxiety, 31*(2), 115-23.

[171] Long, Z., Medlock, C., Dzemidzic, M., Shin, Y. W., Goddard, A. W., & Dydak, U. (2013). Decreased GABA levels in anterior cingulate cortex/medial prefrontal cortex in panic disorder. *Progress in neuro-psychopharmacology & biological psychiatry, 44*, 131-5.

[172] Winkelman JW; Buxton OM; Jensen JE; Benson KL; O'Connor SP; Wang W; Renshaw PF. Reduced brain GABA in primary insomnia: preliminary data from 4T proton magnetic resonance spectroscopy (1H-MRS). *SLEEP* 2008;31(11):1499–1506.

[173] Becker, S., & Schweinhardt, P. (2011). Dysfunctional neurotransmitter systems in fibromyalgia, their role in central stress circuitry and pharmacological actions on these systems. *Pain research and treatment, 2012*, 741746.

[174] Israel Pérez-Torres, Alejandra María Zuniga-Munoz and Veronica Guarner-Lans. (2017). "Beneficial Effects of the Amino Acid Glycine", Mini-Reviews in Medicinal Chemistry *17*, 15.

[175] Purves D, Augustine GJ, Fitzpatrick D, et al., editors. Neuroscience. 2nd edition. Sunderland (MA): Sinauer Associates; 2001. GABA and Glycine. Available from: https://www.ncbi.nlm.nih.gov/books/NBK11084

[176] Chahal, H., D'Souza, SW. And Barson, AJ. Et al. (1998). Modulation by magnesium of N-methyl-D-aspartate receptors in developing human brain. *Archives of Disease in Childhood 78*, 116-120.

[177] Littlejohn, G., & Guymer, E. (2017). Modulation of NMDA Receptor Activity in Fibromyalgia. *Biomedicines, 5*(2), 15.

[178] Romano TJ. And Stiller JW. (1994). Magnesium deficiency in fibromyalgia syndrome. *J Nutr Med. 4(2)*, 165-167.

[179] Eisinger, J., Plantamura, A., Marie, PA. and Ayavou, T. (1994). Selenium and magnesium status in fibromyalgia. *Magnesium Research 7(3-4)*, 285-288.

[180] Cox, IM., Campbell, MJ. And Dowson, DI. (1991). Red blood cell magnesium levels and the chronic fatigue syndrome (ME); a case control study and a randomised controlled trial. *Lancet 337(8744)*, 757-760.

[181] Abraham GE. and Flechas JD. (1992). Management of Fibromyalgia: Rationale for the Use of Magnesium and Malic Acid. *Journal of Nutritional Medicine 3*, 49-59.

[182] Russell, IJ., Michalek, JE., Flechas, JD. and Abraham GE. (1995). Treatment of fibromyalgia syndrome with Super Malic: a randomized, double blind, placebo controlled, crossover pilot study. *Journal of Rheumatology 22(5)*, 953-958.

[183] Calder, PC. (2017). Omega-3 fatty acids and inflammatory processes: from molecules to man. *Biochemical Society Transactions 45*(5), 1105-1115.

[184] Ko, GD., Nowacki, NB., Arseneau, L., Eitel, M. and Hum, A. (2010). Omega-3 fatty acids for neuropathic pain: case series. *Clinical Journal of Pain 26*,(2), 168-172.

[185] Maroon, JC. And Bost, JW. (2006). Omega-3 fatty acids (fish oil) as an anti-inflammatory: an alternative to nonsteroidal anti-inflammatory drugs for discogenic pain. *Surgical Neurology 65*(4), 326-331.

[186] Serhan, CN. (2014). Pro-resolving lipid mediators are leads for resolution physiology. *Nature 510*(7503), 92-101.

[187] Morse N. L. (2012). Benefits of docosahexaenoic acid, folic acid, vitamin D and iodine on foetal and infant brain development and function following maternal supplementation during pregnancy and lactation. *Nutrients, 4*(7), 799-840.

[188] Mills, JD., Hadley, K. and Bailes, JE. (2011). Dietary Supplementation With the Omega-3 Fatty Acid Docosahexaenoic Acid in Traumatic Brain Injury. *Neurosurgery 68*(2), 474-481.

[189] Hibbein, JR., Linnoila, M., Umhau, JC., Rawlings, R., George, DT. And Salem, N Jr. (1998). Essential fatty acids predict metabolites of serotonin and dopamine in cerebrospinal fluid among healthy control subjects, and early and late onset alcoholics. *Biological Psychiatry 44*(4), 235-242.

[190] Ramsden, CE. Et al. (2015). Targeted alterations in dietary n-3 and n-6 fatty acids improve life functioning and reduce psychological distress among patients with chronic headache: a secondary analysis of a randomized trial. *Pain 156*(4), 587-596.

[191] Liperoti, R., Landi, F., Fusco, O., Bernabei, R. and Onder, G. (2009). Omega-3 polyunsaturated fatty acids and depression: a review of the evidence. *Current Pharmaceutical Design 15*(36), 4165-4172.

[192] Yehuda, S., Rabinovitz, S. And Mostofsky, DI. (2005). Mixture of essential fatty acids lowers test anxiety. *Nutritional Neuroscience 8*(4), 265-267.

[193] Whitehead, WE., Paisson, O. and Jones, KR. (2002). Systematic review of the comorbidity of irritable bowel syndrome with other disorders: what are the causes and implications? *Gastroenterology 122*(4), 1140-1156.

[194] Costantini, L., Molinari, R., Farinon, B. And Merendino, N. (2017). Impact of omega-3 fatty acids on the gut microbiotia. *International Journal of Molecular Science 18*(12), pii: E2645.

[195] Fish 101. American Heart Association. http://www.heart.org/HEARTORG/HealthyLiving/HealthyEating/Fish-101_UCM_305986_Article.jsp#.V238SaLcBRo. Accessed June 24, 2016.

[196] Roman-Blas, JA., Castaneda, S., Sanchez-Pernaute, O., Largo, R. and Herrero-Beaumont, G. (2017). Combined treatment with chondroitin sulfate and glucosamine sulfate shows no superiority over placebo for reduction of joint pain and functional impairment in patients with knee osteoarthritis: A six-month multicenter, randomized, double-blind, placebo-controlled clinical trial. *Arthritis and Rhematology 69*(1), 77-85.

[197] Lubis, AMT., Siagian, C., Wonggokusuma, E., Marsetyo, AF. and Setyohadi, B. (2017). Comparison of glucosamine-chondroitin sulphate with and without methylsulfonymethane in Grade I-II knee osteoarthritis: A double blind randomized controlled trial. *Acta Medica Indonesiana 49*(2), 105-111.

[198] Qiu, GX., Gao, SN., Giacovelli, G., Rovati, L. and Setnikar, I. (1998). Efficacy and safety of glucosamine sulfate versus ibuprofen in patients with knee osteoarthritis. *Arzneimittelforschung 48*(5), 469-474.

[199] Pavelka, K., Gatterova, J., Olejarová, M., Machacek, S., Giacovelli, G. and Rovati, LC. (2002). Glucosamine sulfate use and delay of progression of knee osteoarthritis: a 3-year, randomized, pla-

cebo-controlled, double-blind study. *Archives of Internal Medicine 162*(18), 2113-2123.

[200] Morita, M., Yamada, K., Date, H., Hayakawa, K., Saurai, H. and Yamada, H. (2018). Efficacy of chondroitin sulfate for painful knee osteoarthritis: A one-year, randomized, double-blind, multicenter clinical study in Japan. *Biological and Pharmaceutical Bulletin 41*(2), 163-171.

[201] Zeng, C., Wei, J., Li, H., Wang, Y. L., Xie, D. X., Yang, T. and Lei, G. H. (2015). Effectiveness and safety of Glucosamine, chondroitin, the two in combination, or celecoxib in the treatment of osteoarthritis of the knee. *Scientific reports 5*, 16827.

[202] Butawan, M., Benjamin, R. L., & Bloomer, R. J. (2017). Methylsulfonylmethane: Applications and Safety of a Novel Dietary Supplement. *Nutrients, 9*(3), 290.

[203] Usha, PR. and Naidu, MU. (2004). Randomized, double-blind, parallel, placebo-controlled study of oral glucosamine, methylsulfonylmethane and their combination in osteoarthritis. Clinical sParallel, Placebo-Controlled Study of Oral Glucosamine, Methylsulfonylmethane and their Combination in Osteoarthritis. *Clinical Drug Investigation 24*(6), 353-363.

[204] Hill, KP. and Palastro, MD. (2017). Medical cannabis for the treatment of chronic pain and other disorders: misconceptions and facts. *Polish Archives of Internal Medicine 127*(11), 785-789.

[205] Miller, RJ. and Miller, RE. (2017). Is cannabis an effective treatment for joint pain? *Clinical and Experimental Rheumatology 107*(5), 59-67.

[206] Baron, E. P., Lucas, P., Eades, J. and Hogue, O. (2018). Patterns of medicinal cannabis use, strain analysis, and substitution effect among patients with migraine, headache, arthritis, and chronic pain in a medicinal cannabis cohort. *The Journal of Headache and Pain, 19*(1), 37.

[207] Lotsch, J., Weyer-Menkhoff, I. and Tegeder, I. (2018). Current evidence of cannabinoid-based analgesia obtained in preclinical and human experimental settings. *European Journal of Pain 22*(3), 471-484.

[208] Xiong, W., Cui, T., Cheng, K., Yang, F., Chen, SR., Willenbring, D., Guan, T., Pan, HL., Ren, K., Xu, Y. and Zhang, L. (2012). *The Journal of Experimental Medicine 209*(6), 1121-1134.

[209] Borgelt, LM., Franson, KL., Nussbaum, AM. et al. (2013). The pharmacologic and clinical effects of medical cannabis. *Pharmacotherapy 33*, 195-209.

[210] Johnson, JR., Burnell-Nugent, M., Lossignol, D. et al. (2010). Multicenter, double-blind, randomized, placebo-controlled, parallel-group study of the efficacy, safety, and tolerability of THC:CBD extract and THC extract in patients with intractable cancer-related pain. Journal of Pain and Symptom Management 39,167-79.

[211] Romero-Sandoval, EA., Kolano, AL. and Alvarado-Vazquez, PA. (2017). Cannabis and Cannabinoids for Chronic Pain. *Current Rheumatology Reports 19*(11), 67.

[212] Deshpande, A., Mailis-Gagnon, A., Zoheiry, N., & Lakha, S. F. (2015). Efficacy and adverse effects of medical marijuana for chronic noncancer pain: Systematic review of randomized controlled trials. *Canadian family physician Medecin de famille canadien, 61*(8), e372–e381.

[213] Crofford L. J. (2015). Chronic Pain: Where the Body Meets the Brain. *Transactions of the American Clinical and Climatological Association, 126*, 167–183.

[214] Fischer, S., Doerr, JM., Strahler, J., Mewes, R., Thieme, K. and Nater, UM. (2015). Stress exacerbates pain in the everyday lives of women with fibromyalgia syndrome. The role of cortisol and alpha-amylase. *Psychoneuroendocrinology 63*, 68-77.

[215] Toussaint, LL., Whipple, MO. and Vincent, A. (2017). Post-traumatic stress disorder symptoms may explain poor mental health in patients with fibromyalgia. *Journal of Health Psychology 22*(6), 697-796.

[216] Karras, S., Rapti, E., Matsoukas, S., & Kotsa, K. (2016). Vitamin D in Fibromyalgia: A Causative or Confounding Biological Interplay? *Nutrients*, *8*(6), 343.

[217] Roy, S., Sherman, A., Monari-Sparks, M. J., Schweiker, O., & Hunter, K. (2014). Correction of Low Vitamin D Improves Fatigue: Effect of Correction of Low Vitamin D in Fatigue Study (EViDiF Study). *North American journal of medical sciences*, *6*(8), 396–402.

[218] Dogru, A., Balkarli, A., Cobankara, V., Tunc, S. E., & Sahin, M. (2017). Effects of Vitamin D Therapy on Quality of Life in Patients with Fibromyalgia. *The Eurasian journal of medicine*, *49*(2), 113-117.

[219] Makrani, AH., Afshari, A., Ghajar, M., Forooghi, Z. and Moosazadeh, M. (2017). Vitamin D and fibromyalgia: a meta-analysis. The Korean journal of pain 30(4), 250-257.

[220] Wepner, F., Scheuer, R., Schuetz-Wieser, B., Machacek, P., Piele-Bruha, E., Cross, HS., Hahne, J. and Friedrich, M. (2014). Effects of vitamin D on patients with fibromyalgia syndrome: a randomized placebo-controlled trial. *Pain 155*(2), 261-268.

[221] De Carvalho, JF., da Rocha Araujo, FAG., da Mota, LMA., Aires, RB. and de Araujo, RP. (2018). Vitamin D supplementation seems to improve fibromyalgia symptoms: Preliminary results. *The Israel Medical Association Journal 20*(6), 379-381.

[222] Jesus, CA., Feder, D. and Peres, MF. (2013). The role of vitamin D in pathophysiology and treatment of fibromyalgia. *Current Pain and Headache Reports 17*(8), 355.

[223] Jones, G. (2008). Pharmacokinetics of vitamin D toxicity. *American Journal of Clinical Nutrition 88*, 582S-6S.

[224] Holick, MF. (2007). Vitamin D deficiency. *New England Journal of Medicine 357*, 266-281.

[225] Jin, CJ. et al. (2007). S-adenosyl-l-methionine increases skeletal muscle mitochondrial DNA density and whole body insulin sensitivity in OLETF rats. *The Journal of Nutrition 137*(2), 339-344.

[226] Mato JM, Lu SC. S-Adenosylmethionine. In: Coates PM, Betz JM, Blackman MR, et al., eds. Encyclopedia of Dietary Supplements, 2nd ed. New York, NY: Informa Healthcare; 2010:1-5.

[227] Hardy, ML., Coulter, I., Morton, SC., Favreau, J., Venuturupalli, S., Chiappelli, F., Rossi, F., Orshansky, G., Jungvig, LK., Roth, EA., Suttorp, MJ. and Shekelle, P. (2003). S-adenosyl-L-methionine for treatment of depression, osteoarthritis, and liver disease. *Evid Rep Technol Assess (Summ) 64*, 1-3.

[228] Sanchez-Domínguez, B., Bullón, P., Román-Malo, L., Marín-Aguilar, F., Alcocer-Gómez, E., Carrión, AM., Sánchez-Alcazar, JA. and Cordero, MD. (2015). Oxidative stress, mitochondrial dysfunction and, inflammation common events in skin of patients with Fibromyalgia. *Mitochondrion 21*, 69-75.

[229] Sprott, H., Salemi, S., Gay, RE., Bradley, LA., Alarcon, GS., Oh, SJ. et al. (2004). Increased DNA fragmentation and ultrastructural changes in fibromyalgic muscle fibres. *Annals of the Rhuematic Diseases 63*, 245-251.

[230] Alcocer-Gomez, E. et al. (2015). Metformin and caloric restriction induce an AMPK-dependant restoration of mitochondrial dysfunction in fibroblasts from Fibromyalgia patients. *Biochem Biophys Acta 1852*(7), 1257-1267.

[231] Jacobsen, S. et al. (1991). Oral S-adenosylmethionine in primary fibromyalgia. Double-blind clinical evaluation. *Scandinavian Journal of Rheumatology 20*(4), 294-302.

[232] Picard, M., McEwen, B S., Epel, E.S. and Sandi, C. (2018). An energetic view of stress: Focus on mitochondria. *Frontiers in Neuroendocrinology*, *49*, 72–85.

[233] Alegre, J., Roses, JM., Javierre, C., Ruiz-Baques, A., Segundo, MJ. and de Sevilla, TF. (2010). Nicotinamide adenine dinucleotide (NADH) in patients with chronic fatigue syndrome. *Revista*

Clinica Espanola 210(6), 284-288.

[234] Forsyth, L., Preuss, H., MacDowell, A., Chiazze, L., Birkmayer, G. and Bellanti, J. (1999). Therapeutic effects of oral NADH on the symptoms of patients with chronic fatigue syndrome. *Annals of Allergy, Asthma and Immunology 82*(2), 185-191.

[235] Santaella, ML., Font, I. and Disdier, OM. (2004). Comparison of oral nicotinamide adenine dinucleotide (NADH) versus conventional therapy for chronic fatigue syndrome. *Puerto Rico Health Sciences Journal 23*(2), 89-93.

[236] Castro-Marrero, J. et al. (2016). Effect of coenzyme Q10 plus nicotinamide adenine dinucleotide supplementation on maximum heart rate after exercise testing in chronic fatigue syndrome-A randomized, controlled, double-blind trial. *Clinical Nutrition 35*(4), 826-834.

[237] Castro-Marrero, J. et al. (2015). Does oral coenzyme Q10 plus NADH supplementation improve fatigue and biochemical parameters in chronic fatigue syndrome? *Antioxidants and Redox Signalling 22*(8), 679-685.

[238] Saini, R. (2011). Coenzyme Q10: The essential nutrient. *Journal of Pharmacy & Bioallied Sciences 3*(3), 466–467.

[239] Littarru, GP. and Tiano, L. (2007). Bioenergetic and antioxidant properties of coenzyme Q10: recent developments. *Molecular Biotechnology 37*(1), 31-37.

[240] Cordero, MD. et al. (2012). Oral coenzyme Q10 supplementation improves clinical symptoms and recovers pathologic alterations in blood mononuclear cells in a fibromyalgia patient. *Nutrition 28*(11-12), 1200-1203.

[241] Garcia-Corzo, L. et al. (2014). Ubiquinol-10 ameliorates mitochondrial encephalopathy associated with CoQ deficiency. *Biochim Biophys Acta. 1842*, 893-901.

[242] Cordero, MD. et al. (2013). Can coenzyme q10 improve clinical and molecular parameters in fibromyalgia? *Antioxidant Redx Signalling 19*(12), 1356-1361.

[243] Acocer-Gomez, E., Cano-Garcia, FJ. and Cordero, MD. (2013). Effect of coenzyme Q10 evaluated by 1990 and 2010 ACR Diagnostic Criteria for Fibromyalgia and SCL-90-R: four case reports and literature review. *Nutrition 29*(11-12), 1422-1425.

[244] Miyamae, T., Seki, M., Naga, T., Uchino, S, Asazuma, H., Yoshida, T. et al. (2013). Increased oxidative stress and coenzyme Q10 deficiency in juvenile fibromyalgia: amelioration of hypercholesterolemia and fatigue by ubiquinol-10 supplementation. *Redox Report 18*, 12-19.

[245] Zhang, Y., Liu, J., Chen XQ. and Chen, CY. (2018). (Ubiquinol is Superior to Ubiquinone to enhance Coenzyme Q10 status in older men. *Food and Function 9*(11), 5653-5659.

[246] Seifert, JG., Brumet, A. and St. Cyr, JA. (2017). The influence of D-ribose ingestion and fitness level on performance and recovery. *Journal of the International Society of Sports Nutrition 14*, 47.

[247] Gebhart, B. and Jorgenson, JA. (2004). Benefit of ribose in patient with fibromyalgia. *Pharmacotherapy 24*(11), 1646-1648.

[248] Teitelbaum, JE. et al. (2006). The use of D-ribose in chronic fatigue syndrome and fibromyalgia: a pilot study. *Journal of Alternative and Complementary Medicine 12*(19), 857-862.

[249] Teitelbaum, J. (2008). Enhancing Mitochondrial Function with D-Ribose. *Integrative Medicine 7*(2), 46-51.

[250] Flanagan, JL., Simmons, PA., Wilcox, MD. and Garrett, Q. (2010). Role of carnitine in disease.

Nutrition and Metabolism 7(30), 1-14.

[251] Foster, DW. (2004). The role of the carnitine system in human metabolism. *Ann NY Acad Sci 1033*, 1-16.

[252] De Grandis, D. and Minardi, C. (2002). Acetyl-L-carnitine (levacecarnine) in the treatment of diabetic neuropathy. A long-term, randomised, double-blind, placebo-controlled study. *Drugs in R&D 3*, 223–231.

[253] Sima AA, Calvani M, Mehra M et al. Acetyl-L-carnitine improves pain, nerve regeneration, and vibratory perception in patients with chronic diabetic neuropathy: an analysis of two randomized placebo-controlled trials. *Diabetes Care.* 2005 Jan;28(1):89-94.

[254] Sergi, G., Pizzato, S., Piovesan, F., Trevisan, C., Veronese, N. and Manato, E. (2018). Effects of acetyl-l-carnitine in diabetic neuropathy and other geriatric disorders. *Aging Clinical and Experimental Research 30*(2), 133-138.

[255] Malaguarnera, M., Gargante, MP., Cristaldi, E., Colonna, V., Messano, M., Koverech, A., Neri, S., Vacante, M., Cammalleri, L. and Motta, M. Acetyl-L-carnitine (ALC) treatment in elderly patients with fatigue. *Archives in Gerontology and Geriatrics 46*(2), 181-190.

[256] Rossini, M., Di Munno, O., Valentini, G., Bianchi, G., Biasi, G., Cacace, E., Malesci, D., La Montagna, G., Viapiana, O. and Adami, S. (2007). Double-blind, multicenter trial comparing acetyl-l-carnitine with placebo in the treatment of fibromyalgia patients. *Clinical Experimental Rheumatology* 25(2), 182-188.

[257] Leombruni, P., Miniotti, M., Colonna, F., Sica, C., Castelli, L., Bruzzone, M., Parisi, S., Fusaro, E., Sarzi-Puttini, P., Atzeni, F. and Torta, RG. (2015). A randomised controlled trial comparing duloxetine and acetyl L-carnitine in fibromyalgic patients: preliminary data. *Clinical Experimental Rheumatology 33*(88), 82-85.

[258] Chiechio, S., Canonico, P. L., & Grilli, M. (2017). l-Acetylcarnitine: A Mechanistically Distinctive and Potentially Rapid-Acting Antidepressant Drug. *International Journal of Molecular Sciences, 19*(1), 11.

[259] Humphrey, L., Arbuckle, R., Mease, P., Williams, DA., Samsoe, BD. and Gilbert, C. (2010). Fatigue in fibromyalgia: a conceptual model informed by patient interviews. *BMC Musculoskeletal Disorders 20*(11), 216.

[260] Lykkesfeldt, J., Michels, A. J., and Frei, B. (2014). Vitamin C. *Advances in nutrition (Bethesda, Md.)* 5(1), 16-18.

[261] Allen, MA. And Burgess, SG. (1950). The losses of ascorbic acid during the large-scale cooking of green vegetables by different methods. *The British Journal of Nutrition 4*(2-3), 95-100.

[262] Grosso, G., Bei, R., Mistretta, A., Marventano, S., Calabrese, G., Masuelli, L., Giganti, MG., Modesti, A., Galvano, F. and Gazzolo, D. (2013). Effects of vitamin C on health: a review of evidence. *Frontiers in Bioscience 1*(18), 1017-1029.

[263] Seim H, Eichler K, Kleber H. L(-)-Carnitine and its precursor, gamma-butyrobetaine. In: Kramer K, Hoppe P, Packer L, eds. Nutraceuticals in Health and Disease Prevention. New York: Marcel Dekker, Inc.; 2001:217-256.

[264] Hirschmann, JV. and Raugi, G. (1999). Adult Scurvy. *Journal of the American Academy of Dermatology 41*(6), 895-910.

[265] Dionne, CE., Laurin, D., Desrosiers, T., Abdous, B., Le Sage, N., Frenette, J., Mondor, M. and Pelletier, S. Serum vitamin C and spinal pain: a nationwide study. *Pain 157*(11), 2527-2535.

[266] Carr, A. C. and McCall, C. (2017). The role of vitamin C in the treatment of pain: new insights. *Journal of translational medicine, 15*(1), 77.

[267] Mikirova, N., Casciari, J., Rogers, A. and Taylor, P. (2012). Effect of high-dose intravenous vitamin C on inflammation in cancer patients. *J Transl Med 11*(10), 189.

[268] De Oliveira, IJ., de Souza, VV., Motta, V and Da-Silva, SL. Effects of Oral Vitamin C Supplementation on Anxiety in Students: A double-blind, randomized, placebo-controlled trial. *Pakistan Journal of Biological Sciences 18*(1), 11-18.

[269] Lykkesfeldt, J., Christen, S., Lynn, W., Chang, H., Robert, J., Bruce, A. Ascorbate is depleted by smoking and repleted by moderate supplementation: a study in male smokers and non smokers with matched dietary antioxidant intakes. *The American Journal of Clinical Nutrition 71*(2), 530-536.

[270] Food and Nutrition Board, Institute of Medicine. Vitamin C. Dietary Reference Intakes for Vitamin C, Vitamin E, Selenium, and Carotenoids. Washington D.C.: National Academy Press; 2000:95-185

[271] Levine, M. et al. (1996). Vitamin C pharmacokinetics in healthy volunteers: evidence for a recommended dietary allowance. *Proceedings of the National Academy of Sciences of the United States of America 93*(8), 3704-3709.

[272] Kennedy D. O. (2016). B Vitamins and the Brain: Mechanisms, Dose and Efficacy--A Review. *Nutrients, 8*(2), 68.

[273] Biorklund, G., Dadar, M., Chirumbolo, S. and Aaseth, J. (2018). Fibromyalgia and nutrition: Therapeutic possibilities? *Biomedical Pharmacotherapy 103*, 531-538.

[274] Lonsdale, D. (2018). Thiamin. *Advances in Food and Nutrition Research 83*, 1-56.

[275] Alemanno, F., Ghisi, D., Westermann, B., Bettoni, A., Fanelli, A., La Colla, L., Danelli, G. and Cesana, BM. (2016). The use of vitamin B1 as a perineural adjuvant to middle interscalene block for postoperative analgesia after shoulder surgery. *Acta Biomedica 87*(1), 22-27.

[276] Monroe, B. (1998). Fibromyalgia-A Hidden Link? *Journal of the American College of Nutrition 17*(3), 300-303.

[277] Eisinger, J. (1998). Alcohol, thiamine and fibromyalgia. *Journal of the American College of Nutrition 17*(3), 300-302.

[278] Costantini, A., Pala, MI., Tundo, S. and Matteucci, P. (2013). High-dose thiamine improves the symptoms of fibromyalgia. *BMJ Case Reports*, 1-4.

[279] Costantini, A. et al. (2013). Thiamine and fatigue in inflammatory bowel diseases: an open-label pilot study. *Journal of Alternative and Complementary Medicine 19*(8), 704-708.

[280] Mikkelsen, K. and Apostolopoulos, V. (2018). B Vitamins and Ageing. Subcellular Biochemistry 90, 451-470.

[281] Cevoli, S., Favoni, V. and Cortelli, P. (2018). Energy Metabolism Impairment in Migraine. *Current Medicinal Chemistry*.

[282] Colombo, B., Saraceno, L. and Comi, G. (2014). Riboflavin and migraine: the bridge over troubled mitochondria. *Neurol Sci 35*(1), 141-144.

[283] Peechakara BV, Gupta M. Vitamin B3. [Updated 2019 Apr 1]. In: StatPearls [Internet]. Treasure Island (FL): StatPearls Publishing; 2019 Jan-. Available from: https://www.ncbi.nlm.nih.gov/books/NBK526107

[284] Gasperi, V., Sibilano, M., Savini, I., & Catani, M. V. (2019). Niacin in the Central Nervous System: An Update of Biological Aspects and Clinical Applications. *International journal of molecular sciences, 20*(4), 974.

[285] Gasperi, V., Sibilano, M., Savini, I., & Catani, M. V. (2019). Niacin in the Central Nervous System: An Update of Biological Aspects and Clinical Applications. *International journal of molecular sciences, 20*(4), 974.

[286] Depeint, F., Bruce, WR., Shangari, N., Mehta, R. And O'Brien, PJ. (2006). Mitochondrial function and toxicity: role of the B vitamin family on mitochondrial energy metabolism. *Chemical Biological Interactions 163*(1-2), 94-112.

[287] Godin, AM. et al. (2012). Nicotinic acid induces antinociceptive and anti-inflammatory effects in different experimental models. *Pharmacology Biochemistry Behaviour 101*(3), 493-498.

[288] Robinson, CR., Pegram, GV., Hyde, PR. et al. (1977). The effects of nicotinamide upon sleep in humans. *Biological Psychiatry 12*, 139-143.

[289] Kosaka M., Kikui, S., Fujiwara, T. and Kimoto, T. (1966) Action of pantethine on the adrenal cortex. *Horumon To Rinsho 14*, 843-847.

[290] Gominak, SC. (2016). Vitamin D deficiency changes the intestinal microbiome reducing B vitamin production in the gut. The resulting lack of pantothenic acid adversely affects the immune system, producing a "pro-inflammatory" state associated with atherosclerosis and auto-immunity. *Medical Hypotheses 94*, 103-107.

[291] Kosaka C, Okida M, Kaneyuki T, et al. (1973). Action of pantethine on the adrenal cortex of hypophysectomized rats. *Horumon To Rinsho 21*, 517-525.

[292] Ralli D. NYU Bellevue Med Center, 1952. [Abstract]

[293] Kelly, GS. (1999). Nutritional and botanical interventions to assist with the adaptation to stress. *Alternative Medicine Review 4*(4), 249-265.

[294] Ueland, PM., McCann, A., Midttun, O. and Ulvik, A. (2017). Inflammation, vitamin B6 and related pathways. *Molecular Aspects of Medicine 53*, (10-27).

[295] Hvas, AM., Juul, S., Bech, P. And Nexo, E. (2004). Vitamin B6 level is associated with symptoms of depression. *Psychotherapy and Psychosomatics 73*(6), 340-343.

[296] Hellmann, H. and Mooney, S. (2010). Vitamin B6: a molecule for human health? *Molecules 15*(1), 442-459.

[297] Sato, K. (2018). Why is vitamin B6 effective in alleviating the symptoms of autism? *Medical Hypotheses 115*, 103-106.

[298] Zempleni, J. (2005). Uptake, Localization and noncarboxylase roles of biotin. *Annual Review of Nutrition 25*(1), 175-196.

[299] Salie, MJ. and Thelen, JJ. (2016). Regulation and structure of the heteromeric acetyl-CoA carboxylase. *Biochimica et Biophysica Acta 1861*(9), 1207-1213.

[300] Maier-Janson, W. (2018). Biotin-deficiency in patients with fibromyalgia syndrome combined with small fiber pathology. *Neurology 90*(15), 102.

[301] Heidker, RM., Emerson, MR. and LeVine, SM. (2016). Intersections of pathways involving biotin and iron relative to therapeutic mechanisms for progressive multiple sclerosis. *Discovery Medicine 22*(1), 381-387.

[302] Likis, F. (2016). Folic Acid. *Journal of Midwifery and Womens Health 61*(6), 797-798.

[303] Latremoliere, A. and Costigan, M. (2011). GCH1, BH4 and pain. *Current Pharmaceutical Biotechnology 12*(10), 1728-1741.

[304] Regland, B., Forsmark, S., Halaouate, L., Matousek, M., Peilot, B., Zachrisson, O. and Gottfries, CG. (2015). Response to vitamin B12 and folic acid in myalgic encephalomyelitis and fibromyalgia. *PLoS One 10*(4), e0124648.

[305] Tavares, J., Baptista, B., Gonçalves, B., & Horta, A. B. (2019). Pernicious Anaemia with Normal Vitamin B12. *European journal of case reports in internal medicine, 6*(2), 001045.

[306] Tavares, J., Baptista, B., Gonçalves, B., & Horta, A. B. (2019). Pernicious Anaemia with Normal

Vitamin B12. *European journal of case reports in internal medicine, 6*(2), 001045.

[307] Toh, BH. (2017). Pathophysiology and laboratory diagnosis of pernicious anemia. *Immunologic Research 65*(1), 326-330.

[308] Regland, B. et al. (1997). Increased concentrations of homocysteine in the cerebrospinal fluid in patients with fibromyalgia and chronic fatigue syndrome. *Scandinavian Journal of Rheumatology* 26(4), 301-307.

[309] Mato, J. M., Martínez-Chantar, M. L., & Lu, S. C. (2013). S-adenosylmethionine metabolism and liver disease. *Annals of hepatology, 12*(2), 183–189.

[310] Gröber, U., Kisters, K., & Schmidt, J. (2013). Neuroenhancement with vitamin B12-underestimated neurological significance. *Nutrients, 5*(12), 5031–5045.

[311] Eckert, M. and Schejbal, P. (1992).Therapy of neuropathies with a vitamin B combination. Symptomatic treatment of painful diseases of the peripheral nervous system with a combination preparation of thiamine, pyridoxine and cyanocobalmin. *Fortschritte der Medizine 110*(29), 544-548.

[312] Uchiyama, M., Mayer, G., Okawa, M. and Meier-Ewert, K. (1995). Effects of vitamin B12 on human circadian body temperature rhythm. *Neuroscience Letters 192*(1-4), 219.

[313] Martin, CR., Osadchiy, V., Kalani, A. and Mayer, EA. (2018). The Brain-Gut Microbiome Axis. *Cellular and Molecular Gastroenterology and Hepatology 6*(2), 133-148.

[314] Lattanzio, SM. (2017). Fibromyalgia Syndrome: A metabolic approach grounded in biochemistry for the remission of symptoms. *Frontiers in Medicine 4*, 198.

[315] Tran, N., Zhebrak, M., Yacoub, C., Pelletier, J. and Hawley, D. (2019). The gut-brain relationship: investigating the effect of multispecies probiotics on anxiety in a randomized placebo-controlled trial of healthy young adults. *Journal of Affective Disorders 8*(252), 271-277.

[316] Borre, Y. E., Moloney, R. D., Clarke, G., Dinan, T. G. and Cryan, J. F. (2014). The impact of microbiota on brain and behavior: mechanisms; therapeutic potential. *Advances in Experimental Medicine and Biology* 817, 373–403.

[317] Schatz, RA. et al. (2018). Gastrointestinal and Hepatic Disease in Fibromyalgia. *Rheumatic Diseases Clinics of North America 44*(1), 131-142.

[318] Malatji, BG. Mason, S., Mienie, LJ., Weyers, RA., Meryer, H., van Reenen, M. and Reinecke, CJ. (2019). The GC-MS metabolomics signature in patients with fibromyalgia syndrome directs to dysbiosis as an aspect contributing factor of FMS pathophysiology. *Metabolomics 15*(4), 54.

[319] Roman, P. Et al. (2018). A pilot randomized controlled trial to explore cognitive and emotional effects of probiotics in fibromyalgia. *Scientific Reports 8*(1), 10965.

[320] Roman, P. et al. (2018). Are probiotic treatments useful on fibromyalgia syndrome or chronic fatigue syndrome patients? A systematic review. *Beneficial Microbes 9*(4), 603-611.

[321] Tomasello, G. et al. (2018). Intestinal dysbiosis and hormonal neuroendocrine secretion in the fibromyalgic patient: Relationship and correlations. *Biomedical Papers of the Medical Faculty of the University Palacky, Olomouc, Czechoslovakia 162*, 1-5.

[322] Galland, L. (2014). The gut microbiome and the brain. *Journal of Medicinal Food 17*(12), 1261-1272.

[323] Bischoff, S. C., Barbara, G., Buurman, W., Ockhuizen, T., Schulzke, J. D., Serino, M. et al. (2014). Intestinal permeability--a new target for disease prevention and therapy. *BMC Gastroenterology, 14*, 189.

[324] Kechagia, M., Basoulis, D., Konstantopoulou, S., Dimitriadi, D., Gyftopoulou, K., Skarmoutsou, N., and Fakiri, E. M. (2013). Health benefits of probiotics: a review. *ISRN Nutrition 2013*, 1-7.

[325] Zmora, N., Suez, J. and Elinav, E. (2018). You are what you eat: diet, health, and the gut microbiota. *Nature Reviews Gastroenterology and Hepatology 16*, 35-56.

[326] Labow, BI. and Souba, WW. (2000). Glutamine. *World J Surg 24*(12), 1503-1513.

[327] Rao, R., and Samak, G. (2011). Role of Glutamine in Protection of Intestinal Epithelial Tight Junctions. *Journal of Epithelial Biology and Pharmacology 5*(Suppl 1-M7), 47–54.

[328] Garcia-de-Lorenzo et al. (2003). Clinical evidence for enteral nutritional support with glutamine: a systematic review. *Nutrition 19*(9), 805-811.

[329] DeMarco, V. and Lin, N. (2002). Glutamine: clinical applications and mechanisms of action. *Current Opinion in Clinical Nutrition and Metabolic Care 5*(1), 69-75.

[330] DeMarco, VG. Lin, N., Thomas, J. and West, CM. (2003). Glutamine and barrier function in cultured caco-2 epithelial cell monolayers. *Journal of Nutrition 133*(7), 2176-2179.

[331] Berkes, J., Viswanathan, VK., Savkovic, SD. And Hecht, G. (2003). Intestinal epithelial responses to enteric pathogens: effects on the tight junction barrier, ion transport, and inflammation. *Gut* 52(3), 439-451.

[332] Quan, ZF., Yang, C., Li, N. and Li, JS. (2004). Effect of glutamine on change in early postoperative intestinal permeability and its relation to systemic inflammatory response. *World Journal of Gastroenterology* 10(13), 1992-1994.

[333] De-Souza, DA. and Greene, LJ. (2005). Intestinal permeability and systemic infections in critically ill patients: effect of glutamine. *Critical Care Medicine* 33(5), 1125-1135.

[334] Basuroy, S., Sheth, P., Mansbach, CM. and Rao, RK. (2005). Acetaldehyde disrupts tight junctions and adherens junctions in human colonic mucosa: protection by EGF and L-glutamine. *Am J Physiol Gastrointest Liver Physiol* 289(2), G367–G375.

[335] Ianiro, G., Pecere, S., Giorgio, V., Gasbarrini, A., & Cammarota, G. (2016). Digestive Enzyme Supplementation in Gastrointestinal Diseases. *Current Drug Metabolism, 17*(2), 187–193.

[336] Capurso, G., Traini, M., Piciucchi, M., Signoretti, M., & Arcidiacono, P. G. (2019). Exocrine pancreatic insufficiency: prevalence, diagnosis, and management. *Clinical and Experimental Gastroenterology* 12, 129–139.

[337] Laugier, R., Bernard, JP., Berthezene, P. and Dupuy, P. (1991). Changes in pancreatic exocrine secretion with age: pancreatic exocrine secretion does decrease in the elderly. *Digestion* 50(3-4), 202-211.

[338] Ferrone, M., Raimondo, M. and Scolapio, JS. (2007). Pancreatic Enzyme Pharmacotherapy. *Pharmacotherapy 27*(6), 910-920.

[339] Ezekiel, A. and Mamboya, F. (2012). Papain, a plant enzyme of biological importance: A review. *American Journal of Biochemistry and Biotechnology 8*, 99-104.

[340] Abdulrazaq, BN. and Mohammad, TR. (2015). Antiinflammatory and antioxidant properties of unripe papaya extract in an excision wound model. *Pharmaceutical Biology 53*(5), 662-671.

[341] Osato JA, Santiago LA, Remo GM, et al. (1993). Antimicrobial and antioxidant activities of unripe papaya. *Life Science* 53, 1383–1389.

[342] Pavan, R., Jain, S. and Kumar, A. (2012). Properties and therapeutic application of bromelain: a review. *Biotechnology Research International*, 976203.

[343] Bhattacharyya, BK. (2008). Bromelain: an overview. *Natural Product Radiance 7*(4), 359–363.

[344] Castell, JV. Friedrich, G., Kuhn, CS. And Poppe, GE. Intestinal absorption of undegraded

proteins in men: presence of bromelain in plasma after oral intake. *American Journal of Physiology* 273(1), G139-G146.

[345] Domínguez-Muñoz, JE., Iglesias-García, J., Iglesias-Rey, M., Figueiras, A. and Vilariño-Insua, M. (2005). Effect of the administration schedule on the therapeutic efficacy of oral pancreatic enzyme supplements in patients with exocrine pancreatic insufficiency: a randomized, three-way crossover study. *Alimentary Pharmacology and Therapeutics 21*(8), 993-1000.

[346] Ursini, F., Naty, S. and Grembiale, RD. (2011). Fibromyalgia and obesity: the hidden link. *Rheumatology International 31*(11), 1403-1408.

[347] Coskun Benlidayi, I. (2019). Role of inflammation in the pathogenesis and treatment of fibromyalgia. *Rheumatology International 39*(5), 781-791.

[348] Popkin, BM., D'Anci, KE. and Rosenberg, IH. (2010). Water, hydration and health. *Nutrition Reviews 68*(8), 439-458.

[349] Dennis, EA. et al. (2010). Water consumption increases weight loss during a hypocaloric diet intervention in middle-aged and older adults. *Obesity* 18(2), 300-307.

[350] Armstrong, LE. et al. (2012). Mild dehydration affects mood in healthy young women. *Journal of Nutrition 142*(2), 382-388.

[351] Shaheen, NA. et al. (2018). Public knowledge of dehydration and fluid intake practices: variation by participants' characteristics. *BMC Public Health 18*(1), 1346.

[352] Cleary, MA., Sitler, MR. and Kendrick, ZV. (2006). Dehydration and symptoms of delayed onset muscle soreness in normothermic men. *Journal of Athletic Training 4*(1), 36-45.

[353] Riebl, SK. and Davy, BM. (2013). The hydration Equation: Update on Water Balance and Cognitive Performance. *ACSM's Health and Fitness Journal 17*(6), 21-28.

[354] Institute of Medicine of the National Academies. Water. Dietary Reference Intakes for Water, Sodium, Chloride, Potassium and Sulfate. Washington, D.C: National Academy Press; 2005. pp. 73–185.

[355] Meinders, AJ. et al. (2010). How much water do we really need to drink? *Ned Tijdschr Geneeskd 154*, A1757.

[356] Casa, DJ., Clarkson, PM. and Roberts, WO. (2005). American College of Sports Medicine roundtable on hydration and physical activity: consensus statements. *Current Sports Medicine Reports 4*(3), 115-127.

[357] Slavin, JL. and Lloyd, B. (2012). Health benefits of fruits and vegetables. *Advanced Nutrition* 3(4), 506-516.

[358] Holton, K. (2016). The role of diet in the treatment of fibromyalgia. *Pain Management* 6(4), 317-320.

[359] Kaartinen, K. et al. (2000). Vegan diet alleviates fibromyalgia symptoms. *Scandanavian Journal of Rheumatology* 29(5), 308-313.

[360] Donaldson, MS., Speight, N. and Loomis, S. (2001). Fibromyalgia syndrome improved using mostly raw vegetarian diet: an observational study. *BMC Complementary and Alternative Medicine 1*, 7.

[361] Martinez-Rodriguez, A. et al. (2018). Effects of lacto-vegetarian diet and stabilization core exercises on body composition and pain in women with fibromyalgia: randomized controlled trial. *Nutricion Hospitalaria* 35(2), 392-399.

[362] Sureda, A., Bibiloni, M., Julibert, A., Bouzas, C. et al. (2018). Adherence to the Mediterranean Diet and Inflammatory Markers. *Nutrients*, 10(1), 62.

[363] Correa-Rodriguez, M. et al. (2019). Mediterranean diet, body composition, and activity associated with bone health in women with fibromyalgia syndrome. *Nursing Research*.

[364] Ruiz-Cabello, P. et al. (2017). Association of dietary habits with psychosocial outcomes in women with fibromyalgia: the al-Andalus project. *The Journal of the Academy of Nutrition and Dietetics 117*(3), 422-432.

[365] Tian, D. et al. (2018). High fat diet sensitizes fibromyalgia-like pain behaviours in mice via tumor necrosis factor alpha. *PLoS One13*(2), e0190861.

[366] Marsh, A., Eslick, EM. And Eslick, GD. (2016). Does a diet low in FODMAPs reduce symptoms associated with functional gastrointestinal disorders? A comprehensive systematic review and meta-analysis. *European Journal of Nutrition 55*(3), 897-906.

[367] Marum, AP., Moreira, C., Tomas-Carus, P., Saraiva, F. and Guerreiro, CS. (2017). A low fermentable oligo-di-mono-saccharides and polyols (FODMAP) diet is a balanced therapy for fibromyalgia with nutritional and symptomatic benefits. *Nutricion Hospitalaria 34*(3), 667-674.

[368] Linnemann, A, Kappert, MB., Fischer, S., Doerr, JM., Strahler, J. and Nater, UM. (2015). The effects of music listening on pain and stress in the daily life of patients with fibromyalgia syndrome. *Frontiers in Human Neuroscience 9*, 434.

[369] Garza-Villarreal et al. (2014). Music reduces pain and increases functional mobility in fibromyalgia. *Frontiers in Psychology 5*(90).

[370] Onieva-Zafra, MD. et al. (2013). Effect of music as nursing intervention for people diagnosed with fibromyalgia. *Pain Management Nursing 14*(2), 39-46.

[371] Fancourt, D., Williamon, A., Carvalho, L. A., Steptoe, A., Dow, R., & Lewis, I. (2016). Singing modulates mood, stress, cortisol, cytokine and neuropeptide activity in cancer patients and carers. *Ecancermedicalscience 10*, 631.

[372] Kabat-Zinn, J., Lipworth, L. and Burney, R. (1985). The clinical use of mindfulness meditation for the self-regulation of chronic pain. *Journal of Behavioural Medicine 8*(2), 163-190.

[373] Kaplan, KH., Goldenberg, DL. and Galvin-Nadeau, M. (1993). The impact of a meditation-based stress reduction program on fibromyalgia. *General Hospital Psychiatry 15*(5), 284-289.

[374] Adler-Neal, A. L., & Zeidan, F. (2017). Mindfulness Meditation for Fibromyalgia: Mechanistic and Clinical Considerations. *Current rheumatology reports*, 19(9), 59.

[375] Taren, AA., Gianaros, PJ., Greco, CM., Lindsay, EK., Fairgrieve, A., Brown, KW. et al. (2015). Mindfulness meditation training alters stress-related amygdala resting state functional connectivity: a randomized control trial. *Social Cognitive and Affective Neuroscience 10*(12), 1758-1768.

[376] Lauche, R., Cramer, H., Dobos, G., Langhorst, J. and Schmidt, S. (2013). A systematic review and meta-analysis of mindfulness-based stress reduction for fibromyalgia syndrome. *Journal of Psychosomatic Research 75*(6), 500-510.

[377] Goldin, PR. and Gross, JJ. (2010). Effects of mindfulness-based stress reduction (MBSR) on emotion regulation in social anxiety disorder. *Emotion 10*(1), 83-91.

[378] Paul, NA., Stanton, SJ., Greeson, JM., Smoski, MJ. and Wang, L. (2013). Psychological and neural mechanisms of trait mindfulness in reducing depression vulnerability. *Social Cognitive and Affefctive Neuroscience 8*(1), 56-64.

[379] Bennett, R. and Nelson, D. (2006). Cognitive behavioural therapy for fibromyalgia. *Nature Clin-*

ical Practice Rheumatology 2(8), 416-424.

[380] Bernardy, K., Klose, P., Busch, AJ., Choy, EH. and Hauser, W. (2013). Cognitive behavioural therapies for fibromyalgia. The Cochrane Database of Systematic Reviews 9, CD009796.

[381] Goldenberg, D., Kaplan, K., Nadeau, M., Brodeur, C., Smith, S. and Schmid, C. (1994). A controlled study of a stress-reduction cognitive behavioural treatment program in fibromyalgia. Journal of Musculoskeletal Pain 2(2), 53-66.

[382] Menga, G. et al. (2014). Fibromyalgia: can online cognitive behavioural therapy help? The Ochsner Journal 14(3), 343-349.

[383] Yuksel, H., Cayir, Y., Kosan, Z. and Tastan, K. (2017). Effectiveness of breathing exercises during the second stage of labour on labour pain and duration: a randomized controlled trial. Journal of Integrative Medicine 15(6), 456-461.

[384] Tomas-Carus, P., Garrido, M., Branco, JC., Castano, MY., Gomez, MA. and Biehl-Printes, C. (2019). Non-supervised breathing exercise regimen in women with fibromyalgia: A quasi-experimental exploratory study. Complementary Therapies in Clinical Practice 35, 170-176.

[385] Evans, AA., Khan, S. and Smith, ME. (1997). Evidence for a hormonal action of B-endorphin to increase glucose uptake in resting and contracting skeletal muscle. Journal of Endocrinology 155, 387-392.

[386] Heijnen, S. et al. (2016). Neuromodulation of aerobic exercise-A review. Frontiers in Psychology 6, 1890.

[387] Gowans, SE., Dehueck, A., Voss, S., Silaj, A. and Abbey, SE. (2004). Six month and one year follow-up of 23 weeks of aerobic exercise for individuals with fibromyalgia. Arthritis and Rheumatology 51(6), 890-898.

[388] Puetz, TW., Flowers, SS. and O'Connor, PJ. (2008). A randomized controlled trial of the effect of aerobic exercise training on feelings of energy and fatigue in sedentary young adults with persistent fatigue. Psychotherapy and Psychosomatics 77(3), 167-174.

[389] Sanz-Banos, Y. et al. (2018). Do women with fibromyalgia adhere to walking for exercise programs to improve their health? Systematic review and meta-analysis. Disability and Rehabilitation 40(21), 2475-2487.

[390] Gowans, SE., DeHueck, A., Voss, S., Silaj, A., Abbey, SE. and Reynolds, WJ. (2001). Effect of a randomized, controlled trial of exercise on mood and physical function in individuals with fibromyalgia. Arthritis and Rheumatology 45(6), 519-529.

[391] Ortega, E., Bote, ME., Giraldo, E. and Garcia, JJ. (2012). Aquatic exercise improves the monocyte pro and anti-inflammatory cytokine production balance in fibromyalgia patients. Scandinavian Journal of Medicine and Science in Sports 22(1), 104-112.

[392] Hauser, W., Klose, P., Langhorst, J., Moradi, B., Steinbach, M. et al. (2010). Efficacy of different types of aerobic exercise in fibromyalgia syndrome: a systematic review and meta-analysis of randomised controlled trials. Arthritis Research 12(3), R79.

[393] Firestone, KA., Carson, JW., Mist, SD., Carson, KM. and Jones, KD. (2014). Interest in yoga among fibromyalgia patients: an international internet survey. International Journal of Yoga Therapy 24, 117-124.

[394] Wren, A. A., Wright, M. A., Carson, J. W., & Keefe, F. J. (2011). Yoga for persistent pain: new findings and directions for an ancient practice. Pain, 152(3), 477–480

[395] Carson, JW., Carson, KM., Jones, KD., Bennet, RM., Wright, CL. and Mist, SD. (2010). A pilot

randomized controlled trial of the Yoga of Awareness program in the management of fibromyalgia. *Pain 151*(2), 530-539.

[396] Curtis, K., Osadchuk, A. and Katz, J. (2011). An eight week yoga intervention is associated with improvements in pain, psychological functioning, and mindfulness, and changes in cortisol levels in women with fibromyalgia. *Journal of Pain Research 4*, 189-201.

[397] Wang, C., Schmid, CH., Rones, R., Kalish, R., Yinh, J., Goldenberg, DL., Lee, Y. and McAlindon, T. A randomized trial of tai chi for fibromyalgia. *New England Journal of Medicine 363*(8), 743-754.

[398] Jones, KD., Sherman, CA., Mist, SD., Carson, JW., Bennett, RM. and Li, F. (2012). A randomized controlled trial of 8-form Tai chi improves symptoms and functional mobility in fibromyalgia patients. *Clinical Rheumatology 31*(8), 1205-1214.

[399] Vincent, A., Hill, J., Kruk, KM., Cha, SS., Bauer, BA. (2010). External qigong for chronic pain. *American Journal of Chinese Medicine 38*(4), 695-703.

[400] Sawynok, J. and Lynch, M. (2017). Qigong and Fibromyalgia circa 2017. *Medicines 4*(2), 37.

[401] Wigers, SH., Stiles, TC. And Vogel, PA. (1996). Effects of aerobic exercise versus stress management treatment in fibromyalgia. A 4.5 year prospective study. *Scandinavian Journal of Rheumatology 25*(2), 77-86.

[402] Vance, CG., Dailey, DL., Rakel, BA. and Sluka, KA. (2014). Using TENS for pain control: the state of the evidence. *Pain Management 4*(3), 197-209.

[403] Salar, G. et al. (1981). Effect of transcutaneous electrotherapy on CSF beta-endorphin content in patients without pain problems. *Pain 10*(2), 169-172.

[404] Dailey, DL., Rakel, BA., Vance, CG. et al. (2013). Transcutaneous electrical nerve stimulation reduces pain, fatigue and hyperalgesia while restoring central inhibition in primary fibromyalgia. *Pain 154*, 2554-2562.

[405] Salazar, AP. et al. (2017). Electric stimulation for pain relief in patients with fibromyalgia: A systematic review and meta-analysis of randomized controlled trials. *Pain Physician 20*(2), 15-25.

[406] Kalichman, L. (2010). Massage therapy for fibromyalgia symptoms in randomized trials. *Rheumatology International 30*(9), 1151-1157.

[407] Russell, NC., Sumler, SS., Beinhorn, CM., Frenkel, MA. (2008). *Journal of Alternative and Complementary Medicine 14*(2), 209-214.

[408] Suresh, S., Wang, S., Porfyris, S., Kamasinski-Sol, R. and Steinhorn, DM. (2008). Massage therapy in outpatient pediatric chronic pain patients: Do they facilitate significant reductions in levels of distress, pain, tension, discomfort and mood alterations? *Paediatric Anaesthesia 18*(9), 884-887.

[409] Targino, RA., Imamura, M., Kaziyama, HH. et al. (2008). A randomized controlled trial of acupuncture added to usual treatment for fibromyalgia. *Journal of Rehabilitation Medicine 40*(7), 582-588.

[410] Sant'Anna, CBM., Zuim, PRJ., Brandini, DA., Guiotti, AM., Vieira, JB. and Turico, KHL. (2017). Effect of acupuncture on post-implant paresthesia. *Journal of Acupuncture and Meridian Studies 10*(2), 131-134.

[411] Pilkington, K., Kirkwood, G., Rampes, H., Cummings, M. and Richardson, J. (2007). Acupuncture for anxiety and anxiety disorders-a systematic literature review. *Acupuncture in Medicine 25*(1-2), 1-10.

[412] Balk, J., Day, R., Rosenzweig, M. and Beriwal, S. (2009). Pilot, randomized, modified, double-blind, placebo-controlled trial of acupuncture for cancer-related fatigue. *Journal of the Society for Integrative Oncology 7*(1), 4-11.

[413] Kwon, CY. and Lee, B. (2018). Acupuncture or Acupressure on Yintang (EX-HN 3) for Anxiety:

A Preliminary Review. *Medical Acupuncture* 30(2), 73-79.

[414] Maciocia, Giovanni. (1989). The Foundations of Chinese Medicine. London: Churchill Livingstone.

[415] Xinnong, Cheng et al. (1987). Chinese Acupuncture and Moxibustion. Beijing: Foreign Languages Press.

[416] O'Connor, J. and Bensky, D. (1981). Acupuncture, A Comprehensive Text. Seatlle: Eastland Press.

[417] Lam, TY., Lu, LM., Ling, WM. and Lin, L. (2017). A pilot randomized controlled trial of acupuncture at the Si Guan Xue for cancer pain. *BMC Complementary and Alternative Medicine* 17(1), 335.

[418] Lin, D., Lin, LL., Sutherland, K. and Cao, C. (2016). Manual acupuncture at the SJ5 (Waiguan) acupoint shows neuroprotective effects by regulating expression of the anti-apoptopic gene Bcl-2. *Neural Regeneration Research* 11(2), 305-311.

[419] Fu, QN., Shi, GX., Li, QQ., He, T., Liu, B. et al. (2014). Acupuncture at the local and distal points for chronic shoulder pain: study protocol for a randomized controlled trial. *Trials* 15, 130.

[420] Li, M., Yuan, H., Wang, P. (2017). Influences of De Qi induced by acupuncture on immediate and accumulated analgesic effects in patients with knee osteoarthritis: study protocol for a randomized controlled trial. *Trials* 18(1), 251.

[421] Deadman, P., Al-Khafali, M. and Baker, K. (1998). A Manual of Acupuncture. California: Journal of Chinese Medicine Publications.

[422] Schiapparelli, P., Allais, G., Rolando, S., Airola, G., Borgogno, P., Terzi, MG. and Benedetto, C. (2011). Acupuncture in primary headache treatment. *Neurological Sciences* 32(1), S15-S18.

[423] Harris, R. et al. (2005). Treatment of fibromyalgia with formula acupuncture: Investigation of needle placement, needle stimulation, and treatment frequency. *The Journal of Alternative and Complementary Medicine* 11(4), 663-671.

[424] Borud, EK. et al. (2009). The acupuncture treatment for postmenopausal hot flushes (acuflush) study: Traditional Chinese Medicine diagnoses and acupuncture points used, and their relation to the treatment response. *Acupuncture in Medicine: Journal of the British Medical Acupuncture Society* 27(3), 101-108.

[425] Maciocia, Giovanni. (1989). The Foundations of Chinese Medicine. London: Churchill Livingstone.

[426] Wang, R., Li, X., Zhou, S., Zhang, X., Yang, K. and Li, X. (2017). Manual acupuncture for myofascial pain syndrome: a systematic review and meta-analysis. *Acupuncture in Medicine: Journal of the British Medical Acupuncture Society* 35(4), 241-250.

[427] Chao, C., Wang, T., Hung, H., Kuo, CC. and Zi, CY. (2018). Therapeutic effect of superficial acupuncture in treating myofascial pain of the upper trapezius muscle: A randomized controlled trial. *Evidence Based Complementary and Alternative Medicine* 2018, 1-7.

Made in the USA
Coppell, TX
04 December 2020